360 Fertility

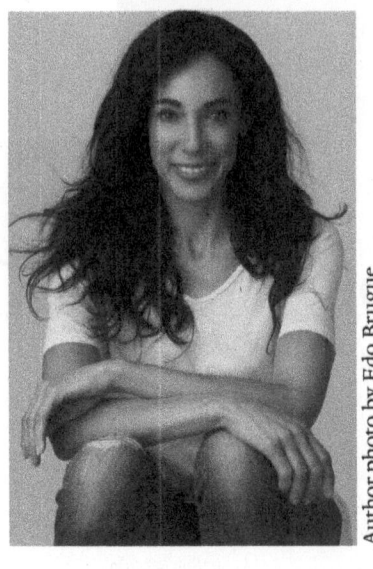

Author photo by Edo Brugue

Liberty Mills is a certified integrative health and nutrition coach, specialising in fertility. In her late teens, Liberty set off to travel the world as a model, however by the age of thirty she was diagnosed with the debilitating autoimmune disease Lupus. Through implementing functional medicine practices, she successfully reversed this incurable disease and is now marker free. Her personal health journey served as the catalyst to pursue a career change and go to study at the Institute of Integrative Nutrition. As well coaching private clients all over the world to treat fertility, menopause, autoimmune and anxiety issues, Liberty regularly speaks at wellbeing events and for corporate clients, and has featured in publications such as Newsweek, Platinum magazine and Natural Health.

To find out more,
visit Liberty on Facebook /liberty.mills.108,
follow her on X @MillsLiberty
and Instagram @mills.liberty
or go to her website at https://integrativeliberty.co.uk/

360 Fertility

A twelve-week plan for optimising your chance of conception

LIBERTY MILLS

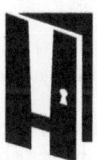

The information in this book may not be suitable for everyone and is not intended to be a substitute for medical advice or medical treatment. You are advised to consult a doctor on any matters relating to your health, and in particular on any matters that may require diagnosis or medical attention. Any use of the information in this book is made on the reader's good judgement after consulting with his or her doctor and is the reader's sole responsibility.

Copyright © Liberty Mills 2025

The right of Liberty Mills to be identified as the Author of the Work has been asserted by her in accordance with the Copyright, Designs and Patents Act 1988.

First published in 2025 by Headline Home
An imprint of Headline Publishing Group Limited

1

Apart from any use permitted under UK copyright law, this publication may only be reproduced, stored, or transmitted, in any form, or by any means,with prior permission in writing of the publishers or, in the case of reprographic production, in accordance with the terms of licences issued by the Copyright Licensing Agency.

Cataloguing in Publication Data is available from the British Library

Trade Paperback ISBN 978 1 0354 2957 8
ebook ISBN 978 1 0354 2959 2

Typeset in 14/19.25 Dante MT Std by Jouve (UK), Milton Keynes

Printed and bound in Great Britain by Clays Ltd, Elcograf S.p.A.

Headline's policy is to use papers that are natural, renewable and recyclable products and made from wood grown in well-managed forests and other controlled sources. The logging and manufacturing processes are expected to conform to the environmental regulations of the country of origin.

Headline Publishing Group Limited
An Hachette UK Company
Carmelite House
50 Victoria Embankment
London EC4Y 0DZ

The authorized representative in the EEA is Hachette Ireland, 8 Castlecourt Centre, Dublin 15, D15 XTP3, Ireland (email: info@hbgi.ie)

www.headline.co.uk
www.hachette.co.uk

To Sooay. It all started with you. I hope this book changes someone else's life, being, soul, like you changed mine.
Love Mummy.

Contents

Foreword	ix
Introduction	1
My Story	7
Week 1. Pre-Work	31
Week 2. Cleaning Up the Present	73
Week 3. Cleaning Up the Fertility Past	111
Week 4. Supplements	123
Week 5. The Four Pillars of Health	167
Week 6. Sleep	177
Week 7. Lowering the Toxic Burden	199
Week 8. Cleaning Up Your Home Environment	229
Week 9. Investing in Self. Investing in the Couple. Making Love, Not a Baby	255
Week 10. Diet	271

Week 11. The New Kids on the Block   307
Week 12. Let's Go 360   325
IVF   336

References   361
Liberty's Trusted Sources   369
Acknowledgements   373
Index   375

Foreword

As a consultant obstetrician and gynaecologist with a passion for functional medicine, I am deeply aware of the challenges many individuals face when embarking on a fertility journey. In addition, fertility is often only addressed when it's a challenge. Fertility is often gender-biased towards women, but now affects both sexes equally. This book gives you golden nuggets on how to support the body to function in the way it was meant to, with a 360 view.

In an era of advancing medical technologies and growing awareness of holistic health, it has become increasingly clear that addressing fertility requires a multifaceted approach – one that not only examines the physical but also the emotional, environmental and even spiritual aspects of wellbeing.

This book, written by an experienced and compassionate fertility and nutrition coach, is a much-needed guide for those seeking to optimise their fertility and overall health. It masterfully bridges the gap between evidence-based science and practical, actionable steps that can be integrated into everyday life.

Each chapter thoughtfully explores a critical dimension of fertility, from understanding personal-health history to cleaning up the past, the home environment and the mind. This is true wisdom. It's a journey of self-discovery and empowerment. What particularly resonates with me is the emphasis on foundational health – environment, sleep, hydration, movement and nourishment – all of which are often overlooked in conventional fertility care. These pillars not only support reproductive health but also lay the groundwork for a thriving pregnancy, a healthy child and the future health of the whole family.

The book doesn't shy away from the hard topics – grappling with emotional scars, addressing the toxic load in our modern environment and navigating the complexities of IVF (in vitro fertilisation). It also brings emerging innovations in holistic fertility care to light, offering hope to individuals and couples who may feel their options are limited.

As someone who has witnessed the transformational power of addressing health holistically, I believe this book is an essential resource. It invites readers to take ownership of their fertility journey, not just through medical interventions but by fostering a deeper connection to their minds, bodies and partners.

Whether you're at the start of your fertility journey or navigating a more complex path, this book provides invaluable insights and guidance. It is both a roadmap and a source of encouragement, reminding us that the road to parenthood is not only about the destination but also about the growth and understanding gained along the way.

To those embarking on this journey, may you find clarity, inspiration, wisdom, peace and hope in the pages ahead.

Karen Joash
BSc MSc MBBS MRCOG ILM PGCert MBBS
Consultant Obstetrician and Gynaecologist

Introduction

Welcome to your three-month guide to 360 fertility. This book will be your companion on your transformative journey to parenthood. It will empower you to take charge of your fertility, whether you're hoping to conceive naturally or by assisted fertility methods such as IVF, with or without the use of a donor egg or donor sperm.

I once faced the heart-wrenching news that I had very little chance of conceiving a child. The not-so-magic number my partner and I were given was 0.7% chance of conceiving with the assistance of IVF if I wanted to use my own eggs. But the story doesn't end there. When I learnt of my subfertility, I was studying to be an integrative health coach and, as I truly believe nothing happens by chance, the day I was given this earth-shattering news, I also started the hormones module on my course. To me it was a sign. A sign regarding what I could do to change my not-so-magic number into one of hope.

Before exploring other fertility avenues or adoption, I asked my partner if he would join me in being a guinea pig, so I could try to coach both of us towards successful conception. He agreed. And so off we went, popping pills and potions and integrating different practices into our modern busy lives. Four months later, I fell pregnant naturally and, two weeks before my forty-fifth birthday, I gave birth to a healthy baby girl. The odds had originally been heavily stacked against us, but we changed the odds and therefore changed the outcome.

What had changed? A LOT. Through meticulous research and personal experience, I uncovered the importance of a crucial twelve-week period leading to the start of any fertility journey. I am now a certified health coach specialising in fertility, particularly unexplained infertility. I am also a trained postnatal doula, because I believe the fourth trimester is just as important as the first, second and third trimesters. Over the past five years I have coached couples and individuals on their fertility journeys, achieving a success rate of over 90%. Everything I did with them I am now about to share with you.

I want to be transparent. This book is not a promise of a magical cure, nor is it a one-size-fits-all solution. Nothing is. We all have a unique blueprint, we all have different jobs, lifestyles, ancestry and history, which needs to be taken into account (but that's where you do the homework in Week 1). This book is a guide that imparts the discoveries my partner and I made during our own fertility journey, as well as what I have learnt in my five years of practice, guiding women and men through their fertility journey to hopefully meeting their Earth child. Over 90% of my clients who have worked with me and done the work on their lives and the inner work have met their child. The 10% who have not are still waiting, but they say they are in a much better position now than they were before doing this work.

As you explore these pages, you'll be introduced to evidence-based research and compelling statistics that all point to the undeniable truth: prioritising your health and wellbeing in the three months before embarking on your fertility journey can make a world of difference. The world of difference in having a live birth. After all, many IVF clinics speak of the word 'pregnancy', but you don't go through all the tests, pills, suppositories, injections and operations just to get pregnant. You do it all to hold your baby in your arms, smell them, see their first smile, witness their first step and hear their first words.

Here, you'll find actionable steps, practical advice and invaluable insights to create a fertile environment for both your body and mind. Whether you're considering natural conception, exploring IVF options or contemplating the use of donors, this guide will equip you with the tools you need to optimise your chances of conceiving and bringing your long-awaited Earth child into the world. 'Earth child' and 'child-in-waiting' are phrases you will hear me repeat. I believe many of you are already parents; your children may have never made it to the earth side, but that doesn't devalue you as a parent one bit. I, like you, have children that I've never held in my arms, but who I will forever hold in my heart. I have been a mummy to many, but people only see the two I have walking around.

Why did I write this book?

I had my own fertility bomb thrown at me, yet I navigated the minefield and came out the other side with not only a certification in integrative nutrition coaching but a lovely baby girl too, who is now a primary school kid. Yes, I'm one of the oldest parents at the school gates, but I'm just chuffed to be there. Over the last five years I have coached many fertility clients, but more and more for IVF prep. I have found that most people don't even know where to start, and the resources in books, on social media and online forums, even from the NHS, are still very lacking, especially for men. With the rise of male infertility, a book for couples is much needed, one that highlights the importance of both male and female fertility. The information in this book is accessible for everyone to use as their fertility toolbox.

Together, we'll delve into the science behind fertility and closely examine lifestyle and nutrition choices. (Are you merely filling a hole in your stomach or your emotions with that lunch or are you truly nourishing yourself?) Further, we will look at Traditional Chinese Medicine practices, Ayurveda and mindfulness, as well as ground-breaking emerging science that has come to fruition in recent years within functional medicine. Everything is backed by science or anecdotal evidence. This programme, these practices, are what I have asked all my fertility clients to take up or explore in the last five years.

More importantly, I'll be with you every step of the way, offering support and encouragement as you navigate this deeply personal and individual journey. Your emotional well-being is of the utmost importance. Don't forget that if you are holding this book now, or listening to the audio, someone else is too, many people are, we are all in it together. Please don't be afraid to speak out or reach out to others or to me.

Let's embark on this life-changing voyage together. It's not predictable, but life never is. I hope with all my heart you in time meet your Earth child, but I think you may also learn a few things about yourself, your family and your partner along the way.

My Story

You are more than welcome to skip this bit and get to the nitty gritty of the book, but for those who want to understand WHY I became a fertility coach and why I wrote this book, here is my story. Here you have MY WHY. The way I felt, the way I was treated, the helplessness, the taboos, the prejudice, the sexism – none of it needs to be there to add fuel to the fire of what can already be a road of hot coals. I want you to know that I have felt what you are going through right now, even if just a speck. In other people's stories of triumph over adversity, we find our own courage, our own hope and we make our own path.

Woven throughout the book, you will also encounter the stories of others – people just like you. These are the journeys of some of my wonderful clients, many of whom I am now honoured to call friends. When you work this closely – weekly, and often daily – on life-changing challenges, it requires an open heart. Everyone who has shared their fertility journey here has done so voluntarily; in fact, a few of them insisted that I include their experiences in the hope of helping someone else meet their baby. I hope that someone is you.

But first my WHY. Here we go . . .

'You may look young, but your insides don't lie. They are still old.' This is what a 'well-meaning' person said to me after the not-so-positive fertility tests came back with 0.7% chance of conception with IVF. Chronological age is often different to biological age. The Oxford Dictionary definition of chronological age is: 'Actual age from birth regardless of development level. Chronological age is a measure of the time a person has spent out of the womb interacting with the environment.'[1]

Biological age (BA), however, looks at the function of ageing in individuals. It is believed that this may be a more accurate measure of the extent of human ageing than chronological age.

'Maybe it's time to get a dog? You are moving to the countryside, after all. A lot of people get a dog who can't have children,' was her response to my blank stare and open mouth.

Or the two lines I heard over and over again: 'You already have a child, you don't really need another one. It's not like you have not had a child' and 'Don't you think you are bit too old for nappies and no sleep? This is your chance to be free.' They spoke as if parenthood were a jail sentence. Or that the desire to have more than one child is selfish and almost indulgent.

I met my partner on a dating app when I was forty-one, two weeks away from turning forty-two. He was four years younger than me (yes, I bagged a toy boy) and the app had accidentally profiled me as being thirty-nine. Our second date was the evening of my forty-second birthday. He teased and asked, 'Could you please stop ageing!' It was funny at the time, but two years later, when we started on our fertility journey, we didn't find the spotlight on my age so funny.

I already had a daughter from a previous relationship when I was in my early twenties, who had grown into a beautiful young woman by then. My chap witnessed the bond that my daughter and I had, and it really pulled at his biological clock. Yes, men get broody too!

Starting our fertility journey

When we started to 'try', at first it was romantic and fun, making sure we 'did it' around the blue circle dates on my app, which meant that I was in my ovulation period. But soon, too soon, there was a dark cloud hanging over my ovulation. It brought a coldness to our union at times. It wasn't about us as a couple any more, but a third person, one we didn't even know we would ever meet.

After around six months of trying, tracking my cycle, checking every time I went for a wee near my period to see if it had come, we came up empty. One time I was a few weeks late, but the many pregnancy tests showed negative results even though my period still refused to arrive. That's the stress of fertility for you. It can even mess up your cycle, the one thing you are pinning all hope on.

When we consulted our local GP for fertility tests, she cast doubt upon our chances, immediately questioning my age and almost laughed us out of her office. I will never forget her taking her glasses off, rubbing the lenses as if that would clear up what she was seeing before her, and asking, 'You DO know how old you are, don't you?' I remember thinking, 'Yes, I think I might know my age by now! I am in my forties, after all.' I hear this time after time from my clients now. This dismissal from medics because of age, with zero bedside manner, even towards women in their mid-thirties. Remember, the number of candles on your last birthday cake (chronological age) does not always corollate with your biological age, and biological age is what I'm interested in.

Back to the GP of doom. After informing me that she was born in the same year as me, she urged my partner and me not to waste any more time trying to conceive naturally and to not even question using my own 'geriatric' eggs. She said it was futile. IVF was the only answer.

Due to my age and my previous child, we were not eligible for IVF treatment on the NHS. Our only chance, according to her, was to go for an egg donor, and even then, it was a small possibility. The GP herself was undergoing IVF treatment with an egg donor at a top clinic in Spain. She, just like me and many other people, had met someone later in life. She reiterated this was the only way to go if we were to have any realistic chance of having a child. She was kind enough to provide the contact details for a European IVF clinic and also granted us both the basic fertility tests on the NHS. Despite her initial comments, I must say she was more helpful than a lot of the general practitioners my clients have come across in the last five years.

So, off for the tests we went. My chap's NHS sperm result came back. No follow-up GP appointment to explain them. The doctor's receptionist simply told him when he called that they were 'within range' for his age, though his motility was low, but that was 'common in his age bracket'. He had just turned forty that year and was told not to worry about it, just no hot baths and to keep his phone in the back pocket, not the front one.

My primary tests from the NHS also came back as 'within range for my age', and the word 'normal' was used once again. I asked for a physical copy of the tests and consulted Dr

Google, as well as any references on hormones in my course resource library. At the time I had been feeling rather unwell for a few months. I had severe jaw pain, was losing weight and was burning up at night. It had got to the point where my partner had taken to sleeping in a different room, as according to him it was like 'sleeping next to a furnace'. Not so helpful when trying to conceive!

I was eating like a horse, complaining of being constantly hungry but still unable to maintain my already slender figure. I was convinced I had a thyroid problem. I repeatedly made doctors' appointments. I was told I had a salvia gland infection, and one doctor suggested it was stress and also asked me whether I have a history of issues around food due to being an ex-model. He tilted his head in a questioning manner, suggesting I had an eating disorder. When all he got from me was a face of fury, he turned to my partner and asked, 'But does she really eat?' Apparently, the word of a grown forty-something woman was not enough for this GP, and they had to ask my male partner to verify. No one was listening to me.

Exploring IVF

So, off we trotted to an IVF clinic in London to see what our options were. The clinic boasted a 48% live birth rate in women of all ages. I know I was somewhat older than most, but they were one of the few clinics in the UK that would actually see us due to my age. Should we not be able to use my own eggs and choose a donor egg, the donor would be found in Spain and the transfer conducted there too.

At the clinic they did more investigative tests on both of us and found that my thyroid antibodies were sky-high. They said in the UK I was borderline healthy with my thyroid function, but in France and Germany, who had different markers, I would be advised to go on thyroxine, a hormone treatment, if I wanted any chance of conceiving, even with IVF. Naturally, I agreed, and I was prescribed 50mg of levothyroxine.

After three weeks on thyroxine, my jaw pain had vanished, my weight was fully restored and my thyroid levels were up to fertility fitness.

Further test results came back, which would determine what treatment would be viable for us. The consultant called us into the clinic to reveal our magic number. My right ovary had stopped functioning and was 'barren' (their words, not mine). The other had a few viable follicles. The magic number was not so magic at all, or even a full number. I was given a 0.7% chance of conceiving with my own eggs.

I felt like everyone was right. I may look younger than my age, but my body didn't lie. I was old, I was barren and maybe

I could not have that second child I longed for. And I was perhaps stealing away my partner's chance to ever be a dad too.

To place this 0.7% into some kind of context, the following percentages are from HFEA, the Human Fertilisation and Embryology Authority (2017 data). They show the average chance of a live birth after IVF treatment per embryo transferred, using a woman's own eggs and partner's own sperm:

Aged under 35: 29%
35–37: 23%
38–39: 15%
40–42: 9%
43–44: 3%
Aged over 44: 2%.

Given the limited treatment options available at the clinic, which only catered for women with a minimum chance of 7% success using their own eggs, we were given the opportunity to explore alternative options, such as egg donation and counselling services to get through the decision-making process. I can't say the counselling helped. Once again, I felt like we were being treated as a pack, not as individuals, and we were not being listened to. I felt like we were, dare I say it, being groomed to have an egg donor. Other options, such as adoption, were not even being thrown into the mix.

If we did want an egg donor, this would mean travelling to Spain, as such a procedure was not possible in the UK. More expense and more stress, to my mind, as I hate – seriously hate – flying and most likely those who fly with me don't much like the experience either. Not a great set-up for baby-making, even with IVF. All that stress on the body would not be the best environment to receive an embryo and let it grow into the child we so wanted.

Personally, I had no issue with opting for the egg-donor route – my primary focus was on having a healthy pregnancy and a healthy, happy child. Having grown up without my biological father, but with a stepfather from when I was four months old, I knew that it wouldn't affect my ability to be a loving parent.

Furthermore, scientific advancements in understanding epigenetics also reassured me that, despite the lack of genetic connection, there would be inherent links between myself and the child due to the way their DNA would be turned on and expressed. The National Centre for Biotechnology Information explains that 'epigenetic' refers to inherited changes in gene expression that are unaffected by DNA sequencing. Though our genetic sequence may not match, with other factors at play in my body, the genes would still reflect my identity as the birth mother, even without my egg being used in the pregnancy.

When I shared the news with my partner, he was understandably devastated. He point-blank refused an egg donor. Even after two sessions with the IVF donor counsellor and me showing him countless studies on epigenetics, he said no, he wanted MY baby. I was crushed. How was I going to sort this? I felt like all the responsibility was down to me.

My partner's reaction to the news was completely understandable when I informed him of our given chance of success with our own eggs. I could empathise, but I can't say it was easy for me either. I felt rather alone. I couldn't talk to anyone about it, as I felt like people, even my friends, would think I was bonkers wanting to go back to nappies and broken sleep just as my daughter was prepping to fly the nest and embark on her own journey of womanhood.

If I felt isolated, for him it was like someone had shipped him out to a desert island and left him there, and he couldn't swim. Witnessing his suffering was a difficult experience. Fertility is a sensitive and often-avoided subject, particularly when it comes to men. There were zero options for him to express himself. Who could he talk to about this? Based on my experience as a fertility coach, men tend to be overlooked when it comes to fertility research, testing, basic examinations and emotional support. They are too often gagged throughout the entire process.

Many of my male fertility clients say they feel that they don't have the right to be upset, stressed or lost in the whole process, as they have to be strong for their partner. The ones who have sperm that's not meeting the markers often feel the worst. It's common for us ladies to share over brunch, 'I have PCOS', 'I'm on this or that tablet for my periods', 'I have fibroids', 'My periods are all over the place' or 'I'm not ovulating'. It's not so common for a man to say down the pub or to the chap next to him on lunch break, 'I have low sperm morphology' or 'I have low sperm motility'. And yet these conversations should be common, with 50% of fertility problems within a heterosexual couple being due to the man.

During that period, we had friends who were going through IVF, but instead of discussing their struggles with us, they chose to completely avoid the topic. In fact, they distanced themselves from us, leaving my partner feeling even more isolated. They were the one couple he felt he could be open with.

I strongly believe that men encounter considerable challenges when it comes to fertility, as they not only face neglect during the investigation process but also lack proper avenues for expressing their emotions or concerns due to the overwhelming focus on women in medical forums and support networks. My mission is to change this, which is why I have included as much information as I can for the men as possible, so they can feel comfortable about their fertility journey too.

Fertility is an incredibly personal journey, and it's often a subject that remains undiscussed, even within families, let alone among friends. Through my work I often see couples who have not told even their direct family members, such as their parents, that they are having struggles with their fertility. Many women don't tell their work that they have gone for embryo retrieval. Instead they simply escape from their desk under the guise of an extended lunch break to see the dentist.

The clinic informed us about the considerable sum of money we would need to invest, and my significant other's mother went out of her way to visit one of the clinics in Majorca, which happened to be near their holiday home. The only concern I had about the whole process was the idea of putting numerous chemicals into my body. I had suffered from an autoimmune illness (lupus) in the past and had opted for functional medicine as a means of gradually progressing towards recovery. I had also witnessed several of my acquaintances achieve IVF success despite afterwards suffering from gut problems and autoimmune symptoms, which made me feel anxious about this aspect of IVF. It was something I personally felt I had to consider.

But my partner still didn't connect emotionally with the idea of an egg donor. Perhaps it was because I already had the benefit of being a parent and I knew my love for my daughter had nothing to do with her being an extension of me – my blood relative – and everything to do with the uniqueness of her. Despite undergoing fertility therapy, he fell into a state of depression and his GP chose to place him on antidepressants to help him on the journey we had set out on to have a baby.

As I've mentioned, at the same time I was studying to become an integrative health coach at IIN (the Institute of Integrative Nutrition), with my focus mainly on female hormonal health. As an avid learner, I explored the resource library and other integrative practices, such as changes in diet, certain types of exercise, acupuncture, and Ayurvedic adaptogens that could positively impact our fertility journey.

Brimming with valuable data and medical research from my studies and other sources in India, Germany and America, I approached my partner and asked whether he would give me three months to coach both of us towards successful conception. I was determined that I could – or at least improve our very low percentage. I knew I could not magic more eggs than I had, but, just as importantly, I could improve my egg quality and his sperm quality. So even if we did not get pregnant naturally, at least we had better quality goods to put in the IVF mixer to bake the cake.

Embracing a new lifestyle

Embarking on our life-changing journey (or should I say 'life-making' journey), we decided to shake things up and embrace a new lifestyle with zest. It was only going to be three to four months. It wasn't for ever. I told him, you never know, you may even keep some of the swaps we are going to make. And he did.

As a devoted stick fighter and gym bunny, I knew it wouldn't be easy to tone down my intense workouts. They were so integral to my being after reversing my lupus and were the foundation of my mental health. I thrived on being strong and seeing myself as a bit of a warrior, but I was ready for the challenge. Goodbye, adrenaline-pumping stick fights and gruelling gym sessions, when sometimes I swear I thought blood was coming up (if you know, you know!). Hello, tranquillity-inducing yoga. (Although I had no clue what I was doing and was stiff as a board from all the weights and little stretching. Downward dog was and still is more of a challenge for me than flipping a 60kg rubber tyre.)

But giving up alcohol? Now that was like asking a fish to give up water. Not for me, but for my chap! My dear partner, who worked in the wild world of London media. For him, socialising and drinking alcohol were part of the business. But still, he did it! I can't say it's a swap he carried on with, but he did it for the time that was needed.

My Achilles heel was my sweet tooth. It wasn't easy to say farewell to sugar at all. Sugar was my little reward, and I needed it during this darn fertility fiasco. Give up chocolate?! That hug in a bar, the sugar rush, the dopamine hit, the energy boost! Add to that the fact that sugar is everywhere and in most shop-bought products. Often I thought I was doing well, only to flip over a packet and find one or more of the dreaded words – sugar, syrups, dextrose, maltodextrin – staring back at me. So, I had to go back to basics, back to home cooking. Back to when I was twelve years old, and I told my single mum who worked three jobs that I was now a vegetarian (I'm not any more). She marched me off to the library, got me a bunch of cookbooks, and said, 'Great, get to it.' It was a learning curve. Goodbye packet foods, farewell gluten-free shop-bought bread. I donned my apron and got back into the kitchen to learn to bake and food prep so I wasn't caught out.

In the beginning, my taste buds cried a little, but my body rejoiced at the healthier choices. Meanwhile, my bacon-loving partner, ever the adventurous soul, dared to dip his toes into the world of fermented foods. Kimchi for a Yorkshireman? Now, that's a comical combination if I ever saw one!

We also included adaptogens such as ashwagandha and maca in our daily routine. Additionally, I consulted a fertility acupuncturist weekly. I chose an acupuncturist that specialised in fertility and also autoimmune conditions, due to my history of lupus.

Many weeks, many needles later, after one of my weekly acupuncture session, I noticed something different. I felt like I had a fever, saw stars, and my stomach swelled to resemble a second-trimester pregnancy. At the time I was working in admin in an office in North London. I was sent home in the afternoon, as it was obvious I was in no fit state to work. I had turned from a caramel colour to grey and was doubled up in pain over my desk. On the tube back, I was seated but I had to grip the chair with all my might because of the crashing waves of pain. A kind stranger helped me board my last train, as I was unable to walk. The South London train station that was my destination was only one and a half streets away from my home, normally a 7-minute walk. Grabbing on to every bin I passed for support and dragging myself along neighbours' fences, I got to my door 40 minutes later.

I called the acupuncturist to see if this kind of reaction was normal. Had this ever happened to anyone else? He said no, not in twelve years. I also texted and called every friend who had had fertility acupuncture, but no one had ever had such a reaction.

My worst fears plagued me. Somehow, the acupuncture had triggered a lupus flare. I cried with pain, despair and fear. I did, however, insist to my partner when he rushed home from work that we still had sex. He looked at me like I was mental. I didn't exactly look like I was in the mood for making love, or even physically capable. I quite firmly told him that it was now or never because I was never going to have those bloody needles placed in me again and I was not going through this hell if there wasn't even a minuscule possibility of making life. So, we did it.

During the days that followed, I was confined to my bed, suffering immense pain not only in my stomach but also in my legs. I disregarded the idea of pregnancy, having lost all hope. I already had a wonderful child and we could always consider adoption since there were numerous children who needed a loving family. Surprisingly, my partner was open to this option despite the egg donor being a no-no.

After two weeks, my period, which was usually so punctual (it comes around 4pm on the day and had done for years, apart from when I was sick), had not arrived yet. I took two pregnancy tests, both with positive results. The sex we had forced ourselves to have after the acupuncture had worked. Yes, we were amazed, but we didn't rejoice or divulge the news to anyone because of the statistics for my age; all the doctors had led us to believe that a miscarriage was likely inevitable.

The National Health Service's treatment protocol was a mixture of good and bad experiences. I now see that many of its ideas and approaches are out of date. As a 'geriatric' mother, I was often treated as a number rather than an individual patient – or patients, I should say, as it was me and my growing baby. It was assumed I got pregnant through IVF, and I was told I should have this test and that test simply because of my age.

My NHS midwife, however, provided exceptional care for both my baby and me, incorporating functional and integrative medicine. Due to my advanced age and previous history of lupus, I had to consult with her frequently. Conversely, the doctors continually warned me about the difficulties of pregnancy, delivery and all the potential complications because of my age. Despite their predictions and statistics, I passed every test with flying colours, defying all odds and expectations. I am not average, and neither are you. No one is.

Near the end of my third trimester, my partner and I were summoned into a meeting with a senior doctor to tell us I HAD to be induced. It felt like I was under siege. She proceeded to lecture me on how foolish I was not to want to be induced. She ignored my partner. She presented me with grim statistics relating to mortality rates and the heightened risk of a geriatric mother with an 'old placenta' potentially delivering a stillborn.

Replying calmly, I said that I accepted those statistics and I was happy for my placenta blood flow to be monitored if that was her concern. Her response was that that was only for women who were overdue. I explained that while it may not be a normal procedure, I had discussed it with the midwife and it was possible, as I only lived a short distance away. Astonishingly, her only response was to laugh and enquire whether I comprehended the meaning of 'stillborn'. She repeated the word slowly once again as if I were a foreigner or hard of hearing. I stared back blankly, using my best poker face, as I was a raging fire inside. I have no idea why anyone would want to rile a very heavily pregnant woman and think they would come off OK at the end of it. I was silent. I felt the supporting energy of my midwife almost holding me upright and proud. As I was not giving in and backing down, she then physically turned her chair and herself away from me and towards my partner, and asked him whether he knew what stillborn meant.

It was then that I breathed deep into my enormous belly and replied that if I solely relied on statistics, my baby would most likely not even exist. Furthermore, I reassured the medical team that inducing labour was not required, as the baby had already engaged in the pelvis, and they would know this had they taken time to read my notes or even ask me. In light of this, I firmly declined their request to induce labour three weeks later. Additionally, I reminded her to refer once again to my notes, as she would see that I had previously given birth to a stillborn twenty years ago at twenty weeks. Therefore, with all this in mind, I was very confident that, at the age of forty-four, I was fully aware of the meaning of stillborn.

I know the medical teams on the NHS don't often have the time or the resources to treat everyone as an individual, but that doesn't mean you as the patient can't speak up and be seen, and thus have a more individual care plan.

A fortnight later, I had a water birth, assisted by two fabulous midwives and the calmness of my partner. After seven hours, a lot of sweat, much biting of a wet flannel and Tara Brach's 'letting go . . . letting be' meditation on repeat, another little girl came into our life and the world.

Four days after the birth of the child I was told I would never make on my own, the journey of my life took another turn. Little did I know that this beautiful new life would not only fill my heart with love but also lead me on a path of purpose and fulfilment. As I took my final test at IIN and graduated on my 45th birthday, I embraced the new title of Integrative Nutrition Coach and decided there and then that one day I would help others on their fertility journey.

As I celebrated my graduation with a refined-sugar-free cookie and a blissful binge-watch of reality TV (don't judge me, no one is perfect), I couldn't help but feel grateful for the serendipity of my journey. My life ahead would now be a blend of nurturing my newborn and nurturing my fertility clients too.

And that's my story. It has led me to this day, to me writing this book and to you reading it.

Some of my clients come to me as their last resort. In fact, most people come to me only when they have tried everything else. One particular woman stands out in my memory. She already had two teenagers but longed for another child and had spent years attempting to conceive. She was going for her eighth round of IVF and she said she needed her body and mind to be different this time. She understood that the IVF clinic could make the embryo, but it was her body and her mind that had to host that embryo. She had been in an accident and her body needed to heal, but so did a lot of her emotions. I remember her calling me after the implantation transfer, saying it didn't feel like the other seven times and she was scared. I reminded her we didn't want it to feel like the other seven times, as they had resulted in short-term pregnancies and not an Earth child. This time wasn't the same as the others, this time it worked. She now has a long-awaited beautiful little girl.

Another younger couple came to me, as they had been waiting on the NHS for IVF for over eighteen months for treatment in their area. The man had a low sperm count and a morphology of 2% that had declined to 1%. We discovered while working together that the man had a varicocele (an enlarged vein in the scrotum), so off he trotted and had a minor operation to rectify this. Today as I write this, I have two photographs of their daughter in my inbox that they proudly sent. Yes, I cried. The IVF appointment finally came through when my client was already eight weeks pregnant.

Then there are others, a small percentage whose overall health, as well as the quality of their sperm and eggs, have improved significantly, yet the long-awaited arrival of their baby remains elusive. While I cannot provide a foolproof roadmap to guarantee the joy of holding your little one in your arms, I can offer guidance on achieving optimal fertility, thereby increasing the likelihood of a successful pregnancy and less invasive birth. Ultimately, my goal is to provide that precious child-in-waiting with the best possible start in life, and for you to be the most vibrant parent (if a vibrant parent of a newborn is even a thing!).

My work as an Integrative Nutrition Coach goes beyond just focusing on physical health. It's about nurturing the mind as well as the body, cleaning up the past, cleaning up who you think you are and nourishing your soul to create the best environment for new life to blossom. While I cannot promise a baby in your arms, I can assure you that, through the process of becoming fertility fit, you will not only improve your physical health but also strengthen your relationship with your partner and, most importantly, yourself.

I am grateful for my own struggles, as they have given me the empathy and understanding needed to guide my clients with compassion and care. And now, through this book, I hope to reach even more souls who are on the same path, seeking hope and support.

Remember, you are not alone on this journey. We are a collective, supporting each other as we navigate the ups and downs of parenthood and fertility. Whatever fertility journey you take, the key is integration – nurturing all aspects of your being to create the best possible outcome.

I believe in you. I know that you are ready for this transformation, and that's why you have this book in your hands. Let us embark on this journey together, with hope in our hearts and determination in our spirits. Together, we will empower you to enhance your egg quality, improve sperm results, and strengthen your relationships.

This is your time. Let us begin this journey towards a healthier and happier you, as we pave the way for the beautiful life waiting to be embraced in your arms. You are destined for greatness, and I am here to walk by your side every step of the way.

So, let's begin!

Week 1. Pre-Work

I believe that making a baby is a little like making a cake. First, you find a tried-and-tested recipe. Then you investigate the cupboards to make sure you have all the ingredients and in the right amounts. Then, if you are like me, you set about cleaning up the mess from the last meal (to be more accurate, you get your partner to do it . . .). Then you get yourself in the mood, maybe put on some music, refresh your mind with the recipe, don your apron and get set!

If baking is not your thing, what about a marathon? You wouldn't run 26.2 miles with no preparation, would you? No, you'd sign up for the run, then work out what your current fitness is, what needs changing and what needs investing in. Perhaps a time frame is decided upon between you and your personal trainer in which to prepare. Certain foods are removed and others introduced, and specific supplements become a daily norm. Your plan is devised to support you not only on the big day, but during the run-up to the big day too.

Just as you need to wipe the kitchen surfaces down before you roll out your pastry, the same goes for fertility. This is your pre-work. This is where you find out what needs cleaning up, balancing and updating in your life.

This is the week we look at your past and the present and put a spotlight on the areas that require a little care and attention. After all, your body, mind and day-to-day is all contributing to your fertility journey. It's not solely about the egg and the sperm. If it were, unexplained infertility would not be such a common diagnosis.

The Health History

Coming from an integrative health coach perspective, I believe that often the keys to unlock our closed doors to wellness (that seem at times bloody welded shut) are right in front of us, but we just can't see them. They are in our blind spot. It's a bit like being in a maze; you simply don't know which way to turn and keep coming to a dead end. Confused and frustrated, you end up going round and round and sometimes end up back at the beginning and start all over again, but this time you take a different route. It's only when you get an aerial view that you can see the whole picture and your path with clarity. You are given the map to the centre. This is where a health history comes into play; it gives you the aerial view.

Most of the time your general practitioner doesn't have time to investigate the potential routes of the maze. In the UK, you're typically given 10 minutes at an NHS appointment to list your one ailment and come away with a prescription to try.

It takes hours to delve into your life history as well as your current lifestyle. Even if your GP did have the time, you may not volunteer the right important information, as you may not know that it's relevant. You may not have even asked yourself the questions or asked your parents the questions I am going to ask you in this chapter.

In this book, I have tried to cover the key areas of investigation, just as I would if you were my client. You ARE my client; you bought the book, you are on the quest. In this case, however, we are just communicating through the written word instead of in person.

I normally ask clients to fill out a health history form the week before we begin our sessions. You may find some of the questions strange and think, 'What does this have to do with my fertility?' But fertility fitness is 360-degree fitness: mind, body and soul. Everything is a part of the machine we call a human.

Please fill out the relevant forms on the following pages. You may well uncover some contributing factors to why your fertility journey is taking longer than you would like. Use a pencil if you would like to gift this book once you have used it.

Women's Health History

A. The Mother Lineage

1. What was your mother's pregnancy like?
2. Did she smoke?
3. Was she working?
4. What was going on in her community at the time?
5. Was she alone?
6. Had she had previous miscarriages?
7. Did she have other children to look after?
8. Was she in the country that she spent her formative years growing up in?

If you are blessed in that your mother is alive and you have a relationship with her, then sit down and have a chat with her. If not, ask other family members who may be able to help you piece the story together. If you were adopted, fostered or in care, try to find out what you can to piece together the start of your life. I know this can be challenging logistically and emotionally. I did not find out about my biological father's medical history until I was thirty (which is when I first met him), but when I did it filled in a lot of missing medical gaps.

B. Your Birth Story

1. Were you born vaginally?
2. Were you born by Caesarean section? If so, was it planned or an emergency?
3. Was there any intervention?
4. Was your mother given any medication at the hopsital?
5. Were you breastfed and, if so, for how long?

C. Body

1. Current weight? (Being significantly underweight or significantly overweight can affect your fertility.)

If your BMI is too low or too high, you may not be eligible for IVF on the NHS.

If they deem this to be such an important contributing factor to the success rate of IVF, you must also be aware of its importance when it comes to natural conception too.

You must have a BMI between 19 and 25 for at least 6 months to qualify for NHS-funded IVF treatment. Most private IVF clinics will treat women with a BMI up to 35, but they will recommend that you try to lower it, due to live birth rates being lower for women with a BMI of 30 or more. However, clinics in other countries, such as the Czech Republic, tend to have a higher BMI cut-off.

To find your current BMI, measure your weight in kilograms (kg) and your height in metres (m). Then use the below formula:

> BMI = weight (kg) ÷ (height (m) × height (m))
> So, first, square your height (multiply your height by itself).
> Then, divide your weight by this squared number.
> For example, if your weight is 70kg and your height is 1.75 metres:
> First, square your height:
> 1.75 × 1.75 = 3.0625
> Now, divide your weight (70kg) by the squared height:
> 70 ÷ 3.0625 = 22.86
> So, your BMI would be 22.86.

If you find this hard to get your head around, like I do, the NHS has a BMI calculator online that is easy to use.

2. Weight six months ago: I ask this because you may have gained weight or lost weight, and I want you to think about what the contributing factors are.
3. Now please measure your waist in centimetres and write it down next to the date.

I have found with clients that measuring waist circumference rather than weighing the whole body can be kinder to the mind, so they don't become a slave to the scales. Also, your waist is where the most visceral fat is stored, so it can be a good general indicator of body fat levels.

D. Joy

1. At what point in your life did you feel best and what has changed?

E. Work–Life Balance

1. How many hours per week do you work, including commuting? Please include work done at home in the evenings and on weekends.
2. Hours of screen time per week? This includes work screen time, TV, social media and gaming.

If you have a smartphone, you can check your 'screen time' in your Settings. It also breaks down WHERE you spend most of your screen time. You may be surprised at what you find.

3. When is the last time you see a screen before sleep?
4. How long is it in the morning before you look at a screen?

F. Stimulations

　1. How many units of alcohol a week do you drink?

How do you convert a few beers or a glass or two of wine to units?

Use the Unit calculator: https://alcoholchange.org.uk/alcohol-facts/interactive-tools/unit-calculator.[2]

　2. Why do you feel the want or need to drink alcohol?
　3. Do you smoke? If so, how many a day?
　4. Do you vape? If so, when and how much?

G. Rest

　1. How many hours do you sleep?
　2. How long does it take to get to sleep?
　3. Do you wake up at night?
　4. If so, why?
　5. Do you wake up feeling refreshed?

H. Gut Health

　1. Do you experience constipation/diarrhoea/gas?
　2. How often do you empty your bowels?
　3. What is your average weekly number on the Bristol stool chart?

Bristol Stool Chart

Type 1		Separate hard lumps, like nuts (hard to pass)
Type 2		Sausage-shaped but lumpy
Type 3		Like a sausage but with cracks on the surface
Type 4		Like a sausage or snake, smooth and soft
Type 5		Soft blobs with clear-cut edges
Type 6		Fluffy pieces with ragged edges, a mushy stool
Type 7		Watery, no solid pieces. **Entirely Liquid**

First published: Lewis, S.J., Heaton, K.W. (1997). Stool form scale as a useful guide to intestinal transit time. *Scandinavian Journal of Gastroenterology* 32: 920–4.

Are you doing a perfect poo daily (Type 4)? If not, why? Are you dehydrated? Are you stressed? Are you consuming enough fibre? Do you have an undiagnosed thyroid issue? These and many more factors can be contributing to constipation or loose stools.

I. Menstrual Health

   1. Do you track your cycle?
   2. Are your periods regular?
   3. How many days is your flow?
   4. Are your periods painful and, if so, in what area of the body do you experience pain?
   5. Do you have mood swings prior to your bleed?
   6. Do you experience yeast infections or urinary tract infections?

J. Food Information

   1. Daily Diet

      Breakfast
      Lunch
      Dinner
      Snacks
      Liquids

   2. What percentage of your food is home-cooked?
   3. Do you intermittent fast or carry out longer fasts for fitness or religion?

K. Miscellaneous

1. Do you crave sugar? If so, when?
2. Do you crave coffee? If so, when?
3. Do you have any major addictions and at what point in the day do they come into play?
4. How would you rate your anxiety on a scale of 0–10?
5. How would you rate your energy on a scale of 0–10?
6. When was the last time you took antibiotics?
7. How is your oral health?

Men's Health History

A. The Mother Lineage

1. What was your mother's pregnancy like?
2. Did she smoke?
3. Was she working?
4. What was going on in her community at the time?
5. Was she alone?
6. Had she had previous miscarriages?
7. Did she have other children to look after?
8. Was she in the country that she spent her formative years growing up in?

If you are blessed in that your mother is alive and you have a relationship with her, then sit down and have a chat with her.

If not, ask other family members who may be able to help you piece the story together. If you were adopted, fostered or in care, try to find out what you can to piece together the start of your life. I know this can be challenging logistically and emotionally. I did not find out my paternal birth story until I was thirty, but when I did it filled in a lot of missing medical gaps.

B. Your Birth Story

1. Were you born vaginally?
2. Were you born by Caesarean section? If so, was it planned or an emergency?
3. Was there any intervention?
4. Was your mother given any medication at the hospital?
5. Were you breastfed and, if so, for how long?

C. Body

1. Current weight? (Being significantly underweight or significantly overweight can affect your fertility).

In the UK the NHS guidelines for a man's BMI in relation to fertility are as follows:

'Having a body mass index (BMI) above 29 may reduce fertility.'

Men have hormones too and being overweight can and often does create a hormonal imbalance.

Studies even as recent as May 2023 have linked obesity to poor sperm quality.[3]

2. Weight six months ago? I ask this because you may have gained weight or lost weight and I want you to think about what the contributing factors are.
3. Now please measure your waist in centimetres and write that down next to the date.

I have found with clients that measuring waist circumference rather than weighing the whole body can be kinder to the mind, so they don't become a slave to the scales. Also, your waist is where the most visceral fat is stored, so it can be a good general indicator of body fat levels.

D. Joy

1. At what point in your life did you feel best and what has changed?

E. Work–Life Balance

1. How many hours per week do you work, including commuting? Please include work done at home in the evenings and on weekends.

2. Hours of screen time per week? This includes work screen time, TV, social media and gaming.

If you have a smartphone, you can check your 'screen time' in your Settings. It also breaks down WHERE you spend most of your screen time. You may be surprised at what you find.

3. When is the last time you see a screen before sleep?
4. How long is it in the morning before you look at a screen?

F. Stimulations

1. How many units of alcohol a week do you drink?

How do you convert a few beers or a glass or two of wine to units?

Use the Unit calculator: https://alcoholchange.org.uk/alcohol-facts/interactive-tools/unit-calculator.

2. Why do you drink alcohol?
3. Do you smoke and, if so, how many a day?
4. Do you vape? If so, when?

G. Rest

1. How many hours do you sleep?
2. How long does it take to get to sleep?

3. Do you wake up at night?
4. If so, why?

H. Gut Health

1. Do you experience constipation/diarrhoea/gas?
2. How often do you empty your bowels?
3. What is your average weekly number on the Bristol stool chart? https://www.nice.org.uk/guidance/cg99/resources/cg99-constipation-in-children-and-young-people-bristol-stool-chart-2.

Bristol Stool Chart

Type 1		Separate hard lumps, like nuts (hard to pass)
Type 2		Sausage-shaped but lumpy
Type 3		Like a sausage but with cracks on the surface
Type 4		Like a sausage or snake, smooth and soft
Type 5		Soft blobs with clear-cut edges
Type 6		Fluffy pieces with ragged edges, a mushy stool
Type 7		Watery, no solid pieces. **Entirely Liquid**

First published: Lewis, S.J., Heaton, K.W. (1997). Stool form scale as a useful guide to intestinal transit time. *Scandinavian Journal of Gastroenterology* 32: 920–4.

Are you doing a perfect poo daily ('Type 4)? If not, why? Are you dehydrated? Are you stressed? Are you consuming enough fibre? Do you have an undiagnosed thyroid issue? These and many more factors can be contributing to constipation or loose stools.

I. Food Information

1. Daily Diet

   Breakfast
   Lunch
   Dinner
   Snacks
   Liquids

2. What percentage of your food is home-cooked? Do you cook?
3. Do you intermittent fast or do longer fasts for fitness or religion?

J. Miscellaneous

1. Do you crave sugar? If so, when?
2. Do you crave coffee? If so, when?
3. Or do you have any major addictions and at what point in the day do they come into play?

4. How would you rate your anxiety on a scale of 0–10?
5. How would you rate your energy on a scale of 0–10?
6. When was the last time you took antibiotics?
7. How is your oral health?

What surprised you by doing this exercise?

Did you find any patterns? Are you as healthy as you thought?

Let's work through it together and see where I can help and ask some more probing questions for where things may need to be healed or restored and replenished.

Why do I ask about your mother's experience of your birth?

Were you fed from conception? You have most likely picked up this book, or are listening to me talk away, because you know that nutrition in all its forms can make some level of difference to the body. Today, overall wellbeing has evolved greatly. Even in the last five to ten years, huge advances have been made in science and education, and this information is much more available because of the internet. Back in the eighties or nineties 'superfoods', 'protein' and the 'gut' were not general buzzwords. Therefore, there is no judgement here; if your mum smoked, partied, ate junk food all day while pregnant, she did what she needed to do at the time. Let it go. However, these lifestyle choices were the making of you, so now is the time to do a retune.

If your mum had to have antibiotics or other medications when pregnant or during birth, this would have affected your mitochondria from day one, so you will need to look at what you can do to improve it now you are making your baby. Why? A newborn's mitochondrial health affects their growth and development, including that of their reproductive organs.

This is especially important if you were born female because, ladies, when you were a baby inside your mother, all your eggs were already inside you! We are forever connected. For example, I was rather a sickly baby, but my mum was young when she had me, she was alone, and she didn't have a good supportive network around her. She may also have partied a little while I was growing inside her. Perhaps that's why I love music and dancing so much, but also maybe why I got every sickness under the sun.

Were you born vaginally? C-section? Was there any intervention?

C-sections, while sometimes life-saving and the only safe option for a birth, do deviate from the natural course of childbirth in one crucial aspect – the baby's exposure to the vaginal microbiome. The birth canal is a fascinating ecosystem teeming with beneficial microorganisms that play a significant role in a newborn's early health.

During a vaginal birth, babies are exposed to a diverse array of these microorganisms, which can help kickstart their own developing microbiome and immune system. This exposure aids in the colonisation of the baby's (your) gut with beneficial bacteria, helping to build a strong foundation for a healthy immune system. While C-sections may deprive infants of this initial microbial contact, it's comforting to know that science has advanced, and we now know there are ways to support your baby's microbiome even after a C-section. However, this may not have been the guidance when your mum had a newborn.

One way is leaving the vernix (the white sticky stuff that coats the baby in the womb) on the baby after birth to naturally soak in rather than immediately washing it off. Vernix is a natural moisturiser and protects the baby against infection in the first few days of their life in the outside world. Skin-to-skin contact is now encouraged for both mummy and the birthing partner, not just immediately after birth but also in the following days, as this gives extra opportunity for the transferal of good bacteria from the mother to the baby, aiding in their microbiome development.

Another effective way to nurture a healthy microbiome is through breastfeeding, as breast milk contains beneficial bacteria that help populate the baby's gut, but this is not always an option for some mothers.

As the child develops, some people introduce baby probiotics that are specifically designed for infants, under the guidance of their healthcare team, as they can also be beneficial in promoting a balanced gut flora.

These are just a few strategies that parents often employ today to give their baby the best possible start in life. However, back in the day, when you were a baby, parents were most likely not given such guidance. I know that, in the twenty-one years and fifty weeks between the births of my two daughters, prenatal, birthing and postnatal guidance has changed significantly.

My first daughter, born vaginally in 1997, had her umbilical cord cut immediately and then was taken away by the midwives to be weighed and have all her vernix cleaned off. I was only discharged twenty-four hours later when I could show the midwives that I could bathe my baby, talc her bum and vagina, and rub her in baby lotion, as well as get milk down her any way I could. My second daughter, born vaginally in 2019, was given to me immediately for skin-to-skin contact with the umbilical cord still attached, and we delayed the clamping. After weighing, we were advised not to bathe her for at least twenty-four hours. I was encouraged to wait for days before her first bathing experience, to enable the vernix to soak into her naturally, and to use only water, with no talc, no creams.

It's important to know how we started off in the race of life, especially if we want to thrive. The great thing about the human body, however, is its ability to repair, recharge and adapt.

Were you breastfed and if so for how long?

No judgement again. I personally breastfed my first daughter till she was eighteen months old and my second daughter only for the first five weeks of her life. Not every woman can or even wants to breastfeed. Many years ago, breastfeeding was perhaps not as supported as it can be today, especially if a new mother was struggling to breastfeed. Sometimes a bottle was given in the hospital by the midwives or nurses while the mother was not even there or sleeping, and she had no say in the matter.

That said, I think it's important to understand the multitude of benefits that breastfeeding can have on a baby's immune system, which extend well into adulthood.

The unique composition of breast milk provides a powerful boost to the infant's immune system. It contains antibodies and immune cells that help protect against infections during the early months of life. Additionally, breast milk contains prebiotics that nourish the baby's developing gut microbiome, fostering the growth of beneficial bacteria that play a pivotal role in immune system development.

The early microbial exposure sets the stage for a robust and balanced immune response throughout life. Research suggests that individuals who were breastfed as infants may have a reduced risk of certain infections, allergies and chronic diseases as adults, demonstrating the enduring impact of breastfeeding on long-term immune health.

It's important to consider how these early-life circumstances, such as being a C-section baby, not being breastfed for various reasons, or requiring life-saving antibiotics, can impact your immune system from the start. Understanding the unique challenges you may have faced can empower you to explore holistic approaches to support your fertility health now. By incorporating prebiotics and probiotics, nutrient-dense foods and self-care practices, you can take proactive steps to optimise your fertility journey despite any early obstacles you may have encountered.

I was born vaginally, but immediately taken away, washed and covered in baby lotion, given injections as soon as I was born and given a bottle (apparently to help my jaundice). Later on, when I was teething, a neighbour told my mum to rub my gums with whisky to numb the pain. I slept right through. When I used to drink alcohol, can you guess what my chosen tipple was?

I use my story as an example of why there is no need to worry. If you fall into any of these categories, have no fear: we will start to address any issues in the next chapter. The body loves to repair.

The Gut

The gut has been stealing the spotlight in the health and wellness world for a good few years now, and with good reason – it's like the superhero headquarters of your immune system. And when it comes to boosting fertility, starting with your gut can make some magic happen. But why? Because your gut is the ultimate multitasker, pulling off a balancing act that influences everything. Think of it as the ring master of a circus. It pulls all the other acts together for the big performance of life. So, what is your gut like?

I'm not asking you to book a colonoscopy. No, the body can tell you a lot without invasive procedures and tiny medical cameras.

Go to a mirror, or if you are at work or on a train or plane, pop to the loo. Take a picture of your tongue with the camera on your phone, the front as well as both sides. This will tell you a lot about your health. I do this with all my clients and then we continue to do snapshots of their tongues at weeks three, six, nine and twelve. This shows my clients how far they have come in their healing journey, as their tongue transforms right before their eyes.

If it is not pink and shiny and smooth (without a few cracks), you mostly likely need a clean-up. That's all you need to know right now. Wait till next week and we can start doing a few things about it.

Tests

Book the following tests at your GP if they've not been done in the last three months. I'm not a doctor, so for each test I will impart the basic understanding of why I believe, as a health coach, these test results will not only help you find out where your body is at right now but also help you help yourself. Blood work is essential for your medical team to be able to help you and maybe refer you to a specialist in that area.

Men's Tests

(Finally, you get the spotlight!)

1. Sperm analysis

If you have not had your sperm analysis done in the last three months, please book an appointment. I know it's not a great experience, but, in my mind, neither is childbirth, so take one for the team, please. There are also many at-home tests now on the market, though not all do all profiles.

When you get your results, don't get fobbed off with 'your sperm count is low and your only choice is ICSI (intracytoplasmic sperm injection)'. If the motility, count or morphology is low, or all of them are low, please go back to your GP for a full blood test to rule out any infections or ailments and request a physical examination of your genitalia. If they are all clear, then you should request a referral for an MRI on your reproductive area. I mean, has anyone actually even had a feel down there during this whole fertility journey so far? Bar your partner, of course. First things first, you need to rule out common fertility issues and be seen by a medical professional who specialises in your area. Don't let the swimmers be left out at sea.

Getting referred early to a urologist is a good idea. A urologist is a medical professional with specialised training in the urinary tract and (the bit you and I are interested in) the male reproductive system. They have the expertise to diagnose and treat conditions that may affect male fertility, such as varicoceles, hormonal imbalances and structural abnormalities.

A urologist can recommend various treatment options to improve male factor fertility, ranging from prescribed medications to surgical interventions. They can discuss the benefits, risks and success rates of different treatments so you can make an informed decision on how to proceed. All too often the sperm is not invested in the IVF journey.

Varicoceles (see below) are a common contributing factor of male infertility and they can vary in detectability. While some varicoceles can be felt and located through a physical examination (maybe by your GP), others may require more advanced imaging techniques, like an MRI, for accurate diagnosis and assessment.

Why are more men not having this simple scan to potentially find a why for their fertility issues?

What even is a varicocele?

Varicoceles are enlarged veins in the scrotum, similar to varicose veins in the legs. Varicoceles can keep the local temperature in or around the testicle too high, affecting sperm formation, movement (motility) and function. This is important because sperm counts decrease by an estimated 40% for every degree the testicles rise in temperature.

By consulting with a urologist and ruling out varicoceles, you could be one step closer to resolving your fertility issues.

Please do make sure that the MRI is done standing up and not lying down, as this can result in missing the varicocele. I have had clients who had the MRI lying down and were told they are all clear, only to go back the following week after I have suggested they go for it standing up and, lo and behold, they have three varicoceles.

What can be done if you do have a varicocele or varicoceles? (Chaps, please do not skip this section.)

It doesn't always mean surgery. Your urologist may deem that the varicocele is so small it's doing no harm or they may suggest you have a varicocelectomy procedure. I believe forewarned is forearmed, so I will let you know what happens. If you want, you can also skip to the end of this section and hear from one of my clients who has kindly volunteered to let you know what it was like for them, as obviously I have never had it done personally.

The patient is typically placed under general or local anaesthetic to ensure comfort throughout the surgery. The urologist makes a small incision in the groin area to access the affected veins. Using surgical magnification and precision instruments, the urologist carefully identifies the dilated veins causing the varicocele.

Once the varicocele veins are located, the urologist ties them off to redirect blood flow to healthier vessels. This process helps to improve blood circulation and reduce the pressure on the testicular veins, ultimately enhancing sperm production and quality.

The entire procedure typically takes about one to two hours, and most patients can go home the same day. After which you would most likely be advised to wait around two to three weeks before having sex again to let it all heal. Following the varicocelectomy, patients are advised to rest and avoid strenuous activities for a few days to allow for proper healing. Mild discomfort, swelling or bruising in the surgical area may occur, but can be managed with pain medication and ice packs. Then you have to wait another three months to replenish the sperm and get re-tested to see if the removal has made any improvement.

I have had many clients over the last five years where this corrective surgery has made all the difference to their fertility journey, and the couple have gone on to have their baby. For a few of my couples, this has happened while they were awaiting their slot for IVF to begin. I can't emphasise enough how important it is for you to get this checked out.

Please do not dismiss the role of sperm in the whole fertility process; its job is not as simple as fertilising the eggs, job done and dusted. Once the egg and the sperm have joined together, the egg is the driving force in maturation, but sperm *quality* is also vital to the process. This is something most doctors don't talk about to the parents-in-waiting. DNA fragmentation of sperm is often cited as a contributing factor in the failure of implantation and early miscarriage, which is why I'm such a stickler for chaps to do all they can to improve their sperm quality. Think of the sperm DNA as a spiral stairway that carries the blueprint for making a baby. DNA fragmentation is when that stairway gets broken in some way, making the instructions all wonky. This can make it harder for sperm to fertilise the egg or it can lead to unhealthy embryos that don't implant successfully or develop to full term.

2. Thyroid function (often not investigated in men)

Triiodothyronine (T3) and Thyroxine (T4) (God help me in pronouncing these in the audiobook, as they're not exactly easy for a dyslexic!) are crucial thyroid hormones that play a key role in male fertility.

How?

T3 and T4 are both needed for the optimal development and maturation of the sperm cells in the testes. Optimal – note that word, it's one of my favourites and one I want you to use with your clinical teams. Often, someone can be 'within range', but not in the optimal range for fertility. T3 is necessary for the proper functioning of the reproductive system and the production of healthy, motile (how fast they swim in the right direction) sperm. If you have low sperm quality, count and/or morphology, it's a good hormone to get checked out.

Your T3 and T4 hormones influence your metabolism and energy production, so they're essential for your overall health and wellbeing, not just your fertility. They directly impact your metabolic balance, i.e. hypothyroidism (low) or hyperthyroidism (elevated, which I found out I had on my fertility journey) can impact fertility parameters like sperm count and motility.

3. Folate

('Isn't that just for women?' I'm often asked. The answer is NO!)

Testing folate levels in men is significant for evaluating fertility, as folate plays a crucial role in sperm health. Folate is essential for sperm quality, DNA integrity and hormone regulation in men. Testing folate levels in men can provide insights into potential issues affecting your sperm analysis report. By recognising the importance of folate in male fertility, individuals can take proactive steps to support their reproductive health.

4. Vitamin D

Vitamin D is not just the 'sunshine' vitamin, as some call it. It is one of the master pawns in the game of chess that is fertility.

You can ask your general practitioner to test your vitamin D levels, or there are many at-home tests you can buy online, or some high-street chemists even do the test in store with immediate results and you can then talk to the pharmacist for guidance in supplementation. The UK guidelines are:

<25nmol/L – DEFICIENT
25–50nmol/L – INSUFFICIENT
50–75nmol/L – ADEQUATE
>75 nmol/L – OPTIMUM (we are always looking for optimum)

Note that when vitamin D levels are too high this can also be dangerous. The World Medical Association (WMA) recommends that normal values are 75–100nmol/L.

In many human studies, it has been shown that low levels of vitamin D have a direct correlation to sperm motility, so this is very important if you are trying naturally to conceive.

Ladies' Tests

Now for the ladies' turn to get tested. I wish I could make this section more jazzy, but we can't get away from the basics.

1. Anti-mullerian hormone (AMH)

This is not the only test for female fertility, but it's the one most people know about. This test checks the level of AMH in your blood, giving insight into your ovarian reserve and helps us to understand your egg supply. Don't worry if it's at the lower end, as there's lots you can do to invest in the *quality* of those eggs.

2. T3

T3 is one of the thyroid hormones that plays a crucial role in regulating metabolism, energy production and overall hormonal balance. In the context of female fertility, T3 levels are important for ovarian function in women.

3. T4

T4 is essential for regulating your menstrual cycle.

4. TSH (thyroid-stimulating hormone)

This hormone influences the thyroid gland's function. Proper TSH levels are needed for regular menstrual cycles and ovulation.

5. Thyroid peroxidase (TPO) antibodies

These antibodies are produced by the immune system and can target the thyroid gland, leading to autoimmune thyroid conditions like Hashimoto's disease (this is what I found out I had when trying for my little one). In women, TPO antibodies can interfere with thyroid function, affecting hormone production and potentially disrupting the menstrual cycle and ovulation. At first, the doctors thought I was perimenopausal, due to my periods suddenly becoming irregular and my body temperature fluctuating.

6. TG (thyroglobulin)

This test helps detect thyroid problems that could affect fertility, such as hypothyroidism.

7. TGAb (thyroglobulin antibodies)

This test checks for antibodies that may attack the thyroid, potentially leading to thyroid dysfunction and fertility issues.

8. TSI (thyroid-stimulating immunoglobulin)

This test evaluates the immune system's activity against the thyroid, which can impact thyroid function and potentially affect fertility.

9. Folate

Folate, also known as vitamin B9, is crucial for reproductive health and foetal development. Checking folate levels ensures you have enough for a healthy pregnancy.

10. Vitamin D

Vitamin D is essential for fertility and reproductive health. Low levels can affect fertility in many ways. It's not necessarily the case that if you go on lots of holidays your vitamin D will be high. There are many contributing factors to how much vitamin D you have stored in your body. Your weight, for one: vitamin D is fat-soluble, meaning it is stored in the body's fat tissues; therefore, your weight can impact its availability and effectiveness. People with a higher body fat percentage may need more vitamin D to maintain optimal levels due to the vitamin not circulating as efficiently in the bloodstream. Add to this that excess weight is often associated with inflammation that may affect the body's utilisation of vitamin D.

Many of my female clients come to me with low levels of vitamin D, some in the deficient range. The levels of what the 'range' should be vary from country to country around the world; therefore, I would suggest that whatever is the 'normal' range in your country, you want to aim for at least the middle.

In women, vitamin D deficiency has been linked to conditions such as polycystic ovary syndrome (PCOS) and endometriosis, so if you have been diagnosed with either of these, it's very important to check your vitamin D levels.

Vitamin D is crucial not just for conception, but for pregnancy and birth too. An American study showed that pregnant women with low vitamin D levels (below 37.5nmol/L) were almost four times more likely to need a Caesarean section than women with higher vitamin D levels.

Most people work indoors in this modern age. I have spoken to clients who work from home and often don't leave the house for days, due to so much of life moving online. People work out indoors, drive to work, wear SPF daily and, when it is sunny, often stay in the shade. Ironically, my clients with the lowest vitamin D levels are often in the hottest countries.

So please do add this key player to your list of tests to get done.

Once you have your results, you can jump to the supplement section and find out how best to top up.

11. Ferritin

Ferritin stores iron in your body, which is important for fertility. Testing ferritin levels helps determine if you have enough iron for optimal reproductive health.

Understanding Assisted Fertility

Remember that not all IVF is equal, and not all IVF will suit all parties. There are a number of different IVF processes. So, let's decode them and then you can feel more empowered to decide with your medical team or choose a medical team that will use a process you feel is more suited to your individual circumstances.

Let's go back to the beginning, back to when I was four years old and the first IVF baby in the UK was born in 1978. That type of IVF would be considered today as 'natural IVF'. More common now is what I call 'full-throttle IVF'. So, what is the difference?

If you are considering IVF in the UK, HFEA[5] is a good place to start getting familiar with terms, phrases and procedures. HFEA is a valuable platform because it provides comprehensive information and guidance on all aspects of fertility treatment, including the latest regulations, success rates and patient rights.

Another great website to check out for clinic reviews and up-to-date policies is Fertility Mapper.[6] This is a platform where people on a TTC (trying to conceive) journey can compare different fertility clinics in the UK based on factors such as success rates, services offered, patient reviews and location. This can help with what can be a daunting choice of where to start when it comes to choosing a clinic for IVF treatment. The platform also includes a cost estimator tool that helps individuals estimate the potential costs associated with egg-freezing and IVF treatment, including consultation fees, medication, procedures and additional services.

HFEA's definition of types of IVF:

IVF

Usually in IVF, the woman takes fertility hormones to stimulate the ovaries to produce several eggs. The eggs are then collected and mixed with sperm in a laboratory. I call this process 'full throttle' IVF because it can be very taxing on the woman's body and especially her mind, as the hormone overload is like nothing she has experienced before.

I have had clients who have found this type of stimulation personally so challenging they have gone as far as pausing their protocol without even getting to the egg retrieval stage. 'Full throttle' IVF does traditionally get a high volume of eggs; however, those eggs in general are of lower quality than natural cycle or mild stimulation IVF.

There are also options with less medication or no medication at all.

Natural cycle IVF

Natural cycle IVF involves no fertility drugs at all. The one egg you release as part of your normal monthly cycle is taken and mixed with sperm, as with conventional IVF. You'll then continue with IVF treatment as normal. As your ovaries aren't being stimulated, you can try again sooner than with standard IVF, if you wish.

Mild stimulation IVF

With mild stimulation IVF, you receive a lower dose of fertility drugs over a shorter period of time than with standard IVF. That reduces your treatment time by about two weeks and means you avoid a lot of the unpleasant side effects from the drugs.

IVM (In Vitro Maturation)

Normally in IVF you'll be given a hormone to help your eggs mature before they're removed and fertilised. In IVM, your eggs are removed while they're immature and allowed to mature in the lab, meaning you don't have to take any hormones. You'll most likely have IVM if you're having intracytoplasmic sperm injection (ICSI), a type of fertility treatment used when there's a male infertility factor.

Many doctors are now leaning towards natural cycle IVF with women over thirty-five, as there is an increasing focus on: 'Let the body do what the body does', as Wim Hoff puts it, or in this case, 'Let the ovaries do what the ovaries do.' This way the ovaries have more opportunity to select the 'Queen Bee' egg.

How do the ovaries normally select the 'Queen Bee' egg and how often?

Most women of optimum fertile age in a natural cycle (with no stimulation) will release around three to four 'Queen Bee' eggs a year. However, as we age, this can drop to maybe one or two 'Queen Bee' eggs a year.

I always advise my clients to ask themselves and their clinic what type of IVF will be most beneficial for them and their family, not just the statistics. To me it's NOT a numbers game, as many doctors say; it's not a lottery, it's science and nature working together to find the 'Queen Bee' egg or eggs. After all, like anything, it's about the quality not the quantity. But I do recognise that some ladies need to produce more eggs to ensure a high-quality egg, because we don't produce as many good-quality eggs as we age. Like I say, fertility health is like all health and should be bio-individual, or bio-couple in most cases.

Now you have done the groundwork, next week you can pick up some tools and start a spring clean.

> 'I signed up for Liberty's programme to prepare for my fertility journey. At the time, I hadn't even considered taking detailed blood work. Thanks to Liberty's guidance, I discovered I had a severe vitamin D deficiency, something I didn't realise could impact my hormones and fertility. She recommended an infusion, which helped boost my levels much faster than pills would have, making a noticeable difference to my energy and overall vitality!'
>
> Margarida

> 'I was feeling frustrated because I had "unexplained" fertility and was under the impression that neither my GP

nor my gynaecologist were too worried or bothered by this. But Liberty encouraged me to get deeper thyroid testing, as she was concerned that this was what may be contributing to my infertility. I booked in with an endocrinologist like she suggested and I was diagnosed with Graves' disease, which is an obstacle to conceiving. Liberty truly is a champion when it comes to taking a holistic view of the individual and fighting for you (in my case consistently pushing me to follow up and seek better treatment and responses in respect of my blood work). She has massively changed my mindset from where I was at the beginning of our journey together. I feel like she has given me back my positivity and drive, and for that I am truly grateful.'

Michelle

Week 2. Cleaning Up the Present

Numerous research studies have consistently highlighted the paramount importance of prioritising health before embarking on IVF, or any fertility journey, for that matter. Whether you opt for natural cycle IVF, mild stimulation IVF, or the full throttle IVF with your own eggs or an egg donor or sperm donor, dedicating at least twelve weeks (hence why you have this book in your hands) to improving your health prior to IVF can significantly enhance your chances of a successful outcome.

What the people in white coats say:

A study published in *Fertility* and *Sterility* showed that women who participate in a mind/body program for stress reduction while undergoing IVF treatment have a significantly higher pregnancy rate than those who do not (52 per cent versus 20 per cent).[7]

IVF has revolutionised the field of reproductive medicine and given the gift of life and parenthood to many by providing a solution for couples struggling with infertility, helping them to conceive their child. However, despite advancements in technology and techniques, the success rates of IVF still remain relatively low.

Why is this?

One of the significant challenges faced during IVF is the failure of implantation. This is where most IVF cycles that are unsuccessful come to a halt. What happens is that the embryo fails to attach and establish a pregnancy in the uterus. Often the treatment only results in a chemical pregnancy. The average rounds of IVF in the UK before a live birth obviously varies according to age, but it is often reported that most individuals and couples undergo two or three rounds of IVF before success.

This failure of implantation can be influenced by a multitude of factors. Two prominent factors are environmental and biological stresses.

Environmental factors encompass external conditions and influences that impact the success of implantation, while biological factors involve genetic and physiological aspects of both the embryo (the egg and sperm quality) and not only the woman's reproductive system, but the woman's whole-body system. Understanding the contribution of these environmental and biological factors is crucial to understanding the complexities of implantation and improving the efficiency of IVF treatments and natural conception.

This is where Week 2 comes into its own. It's all about giving the sperm, the egg and the body where the embryo or embryos will reside the best chance possible by lowering the contributing factors that can influence the failure of implantation and limit the growth and development of the baby.

The Tongue

I chose to discuss the tongue first because, hopefully, all of you, just like me, brush your teeth each morning.

Let's look at those three images you took last week on your phone. What did you find? A yellow coating? A white coating? Bumps? Dents? Cracks? These are all clues that your body is giving you regarding what needs help and attention.

I love a tongue investigation, as it's something you can look at every morning to guide you on how to eat, sleep, breathe and move that day. Some Ayurvedic cleanse retreats even get you to stick your tongue out each night for the doctor or wellness practitioner so they can dictate what you will eat and drink the next day and what bespoke treatments you will require.

I like it because it's a check-in you can refer to very easily. And if you commit to at least half of the work on the following pages, you will see a difference for sure. A lot of my clients are often blown away by the improvement by Week 3.

Indentations on the side of the tongue

These side indentations are most likely an indication you are grinding your teeth or clenching your jaw at night, or both. More often than not, we can't take away our stresses about work, money, worries about the state of the world, influenced by the news, our fertility, the number of baby showers we seem to have been invited to lately. But we can work with our body and work with how we respond to those stressors.

Establishing a bedtime routine will help with this. Yes, just like when you were a child. Preparing to go to bed is the perfect antidote to worries and stresses.

Start by switching off your phone 90 minutes before bed (i.e. ninety before nightie). No screens, especially in the bedroom. Stop your social media scrolling and instead take a bath, give yourself or your partner a massage (a navel massage is a lovely way to end the day; I will explain this later), read a book, write in a journal, play cards . . . you could even engage in sex for sex's sake, not just because the app tells you to.

If you still feel tense, write down three things that you achieved that day and three things that you are grateful for. If your head is still running amok, then just free-write, i.e. simply get a paper and pen and write what's on your mind. It doesn't matter how incoherent and disjointed it may be; get it out of your head and onto the page.

Like any poison, it's better out than in. It's like my stepdad used to say, 'Never go to bed on an argument.' He and my mother divorced when I was eight years old, but I never heard them raise their voices with each other and I believe that was good for everyone's wellbeing. I take this one step further with 'Never go to bed on an argument, even if that argument is with yourself.' Our shadow voice that's often at its loudest at night is the one we need to crowd out. I have a piece of homework just for this coming up. 'Woulda, coulda, shoulda' is bad for sleep, bad for your gut and bad for your hormones.

A yellow coating

Candida is an imbalance in the body. It's not just down to diet, it can be stress too. Too much sugar can lead to candida overgrowth, so look at where sugar could be hiding in your diet and step away. One of my clients reduced high-fructose fruits and removed bread from her diet and replaced them with more nutrient-dense foods. In two weeks, her white coating decreased by 75%. You could also look at doing a week's candida cleanse with some oregano oil. The stuff is fiery, so make sure you read the instructions carefully and follow them to a T, and store it away from any small children in the house as well as making sure you wash your hands thoroughly after use. Let's just say you don't want to get it on your hands and go for a wee after, as I need you to look after your genitalia.

Alcohol

I have found that since backing away from social drinking (I never drank at home), alcohol really is the only drug on the planet you have to justify to people that you don't take . . .

In my opinion, for this fertility prep time, you should not go near alcohol. STOP. Whatever you put inside you goes into making your baby. At this moment, it's about creating the blueprint for your child. While there are numerous factors at play – some genetic, some environmental – let's give you and your child the best chance by removing what hinders that and replacing it with what helps.

I know you know someone who drinks like a fish and has no problem producing children. I know every country around the world has different 'safe' levels of alcohol consumption when trying to conceive and when pregnant. My theory is that number is and should always be ZERO! If the WHO (World Health Organization) says there is no safe level of alcohol consumption in general, then, as far as I am concerned, there is no safe level for fertility fitness. If you need help, and you might, please don't hesitate to seek it. One thing I've learnt on my own wellness journey is that it's OK to ask for help. Your GP can be a great primary resource, as can organisations like The Samaritans or Alcoholics Anonymous. For me, giving up alcohol was easy, but I know that for many people it's not. That doesn't necessarily mean you have an alcohol problem; it's because alcohol is intricately woven into our social lives, work culture and much of adult life.

If you would not give it to your baby or child, don't give it to yourself. Simple.

Over the next twelve weeks, think:

Would I feed my baby this?

Would I let my baby drink this fizzy drink?

Should I give my baby a fourth coffee?

Would I let my child skip breakfast?

Is it OK to let my toddler eat lunch at their school desk, while working on a laptop and scrolling on their iPad?

Would I?

Would I?

More often than not your answer will be 'NO'.

So, it's a NO for you too.

Everything you eat and drink from now on goes into the making of your child.

Yes, I do think it needs repeating, as often I have clients who say things like, 'My mum says it's Christmas and it's only one', or 'I have a stag do, leaving do, christening, baby shower . . .' I get why you may want to drink, but in the end, it's only going to deplete the body.

If those two beers or those two glasses of fizz at a wedding have any negative effects on your body, you don't want it in there. It's not just that the alcohol is a toxin, it's also about what the alcohol leads to and what it also takes from you.

Did you know that when we drink even one glass of alcohol, we lessen our quality of sleep? The more alcohol we drink, the more our REM sleep is reduced. REM (rapid eye movement) sleep is the sweet spot of your sleep. It's a vital stage and, to my mind, a precious part of the sleep cycle because it's in this phase that your body works to repair and regenerate your cells. REM sleep typically makes up about 20–25% of total sleep time, or roughly 90 minutes to 2 hours of what I hope is your typical 7–9 hours' sleep a night.

You may think, 'I need a few drinks to take the edge off a crazy week. A couple of glasses of wine will help me wind down or even get in the mood for sex.' Yes, it may tick these boxes, but while doing so it's robbing you of the best source of nutrition that money can't buy, which is sleep.

Sleepfoundation.org reveals the following and it's rather enlightening:

Low amounts of alcohol: Having fewer than two servings of alcohol per day for men or one serving per day for women decreased sleep quality by 9.3%.

Moderate amounts of alcohol: Having two servings of alcohol per day for men or one serving per day for women decreased sleep quality by 24%.

High amounts of alcohol: Having more than two servings of alcohol per day for men or one serving per day for women decreased sleep quality by 39.2%.

Think about it: after two or three glasses of wine or a few beers you are more likely to socially vape, smoke, eat junk food, or watch 'just another episode' of whatever show you are bingeing on, and the next thing you know you are no longer going to bed at 10.30pm on Saturday night, but 1.30am on Sunday morning.

From your body's perspective, you basically got in the car, drove to the airport, hopped on a plane and jumped to a different time zone. If you live in the UK, it's like you got on a plane and then woke up in Nairobi; push it to one more binge-watched episode and you are in Dubai.

Even a small time-zone change such as this can disturb your sleep pattern for days, cause irregular bowel movements and even cause constipation. And if you did this often, ladies, you would see a shift in your menstrual cycle or the timing and severity of symptoms.

If you fall off the wagon, as many of my clients do within the first three weeks, it's OK. But it also means that, just as in the game of Monopoly, you're back to square one and you do not collect £200. If you drink, go back to Week 1, please. You will thank yourself for it; you may even thank me.

Men – research suggests that even small amounts of alcohol can have a profound impact on male fertility. Several clinical studies have pointed out the negative effects of alcohol consumption on sperm quality and quantity. For instance, a 2014 study published in *BMJ Open* found that drinking as little as five units of alcohol per week could reduce sperm quality. The study examined 1,200 Danish men between the ages of 18 and 28.[8]

Furthermore, alcohol has been linked to disrupted hormone production, specifically a decrease in testosterone levels, which can further impair fertility. These clinical findings highlight that even small amounts of alcohol can have a detrimental impact on male fertility by compromising sperm quantity and quality and hormonal balance.

In women, alcohol can disrupt the delicate hormonal balance required for fertility. It can interfere with the regularity of menstrual cycles and cause hormonal imbalances, affecting ovulation. It has also been found to have a negative impact on ovarian function. It reduces the number of eggs available for fertilisation and can also decrease the quality of the eggs, leading to a decreased likelihood of successful conception.

Implantation issues: Alcohol consumption can affect the implantation process, when the fertilised embryo attaches itself to the uterine lining. Research suggests that alcohol intake can impair the development of the lining, making it less receptive for the embryo to implant successfully.

Follicle development: Alcohol can hinder the process of follicle development, which is necessary for the optimal growth and maturation of eggs. This can result in a reduced number of high-quality eggs available for IVF procedures.

Clinical data and research studies have consistently indicated the harmful effects of alcohol on female fertility. For example, a study published in the *British Medical Journal* found that even moderate alcohol consumption (five or more drinks per week) could significantly reduce the success rate of IVF cycles.

So, what do you do when out and about?

Top tips:

1. Tell people you are on a health kick. Or if you feel comfortable, be honest and say that you are trying to conceive.
2. Simply remove and replace. There are a lot of alcohol-free spirits and wines out there, and there are even some very good alcohol-free and gluten-free beers too.
3. If people say 'Just have one, it won't hurt, live a little!' my favourite reply is, 'No, thank you, I don't need one, I actually want to live a lot!' This normally shuts people up.
4. If you're going to a party, take an alcohol-free drink or two. I take a ginger non-alcoholic aperitif. It's in a pretty bottle and I normally have to take two because everyone wants to try it. It gets people talking and takes the

attention off me and why I don't drink and moves it onto the drink itself.
5. Change the location of where you meet friends. Instead of the pub or bar, try a dance class, a sport, a walk or an event. Move the time of day you meet your friends to the early afternoon rather than the evening.

Cigarettes (this also includes passive smoking)

Did you know that cigarettes contain more than 7,000 chemicals that can have a detrimental effect on fertility for both women and men? But how exactly does smoking impact fertility?

For women, smoking can damage the eggs and make it harder for them to be fertilised. It can also lead to early menopause and an increased risk of ectopic pregnancy and miscarriage.

For men, smoking can cause a decrease in sperm count, motility and quality, making it more difficult for them to fertilise an egg. Smoking has also been linked to erectile dysfunction and an increased risk of birth defects in your child-in-waiting.

Please contact your GP if you need support giving up smoking. The pharmacy often has support too.

There are also some great apps out there, such as the Reveri hypnosis app,[9] which comes with a free seven-day trial, as well as Adam Cox's hypnosis sessions[10] and Allen Carr's Easyway programmes.[11]

Vaping

As a health coach, I am mortified that the guidance from Public Health England and the NHS over the last few years has been that vaping is a healthy alternative to smoking. The only healthy alternative to smoking is not smoking. Absolutely NOT vaping.

Vapes contain over 2,000 chemicals; yes, this is 5,000 less than cigarettes. However, think about this: currently, at the time of writing, in England, Wales and Scotland, there is no specific law that prohibits the use of e-cigarettes indoors in public spaces.

Therefore, think of all the places you are able to vape, but not smoke a cigarette. Add to this, vaping is more socially accepted and by some even considered healthy – to my horror, vapes are even sold in some 'health stores'. Overall, you will likely be vaping more often than if you were having a cigarette, and therefore the chemicals will mount up.

For men, vaping can lead to decreased sperm count and

motility, which can make it more difficult to conceive. With the *British Medical Journal* stating that there has been 'a genuine decline in semen quality over the past fifty years',[12] the rise of vaping is something to consider as a contributing factor.

In 2020, a Danish study found men who vaped had lower sperm counts,[13] while an earlier University College London study found chemicals in e-cigarette flavourings could make sperm slower swimmers.[14] In women, vaping can interfere with the development of healthy eggs and can also affect the implantation of a fertilised egg in the uterus.

Another study found that 'exposure to e-liquid, with or without nicotine, resulted in a marked decrease in circulating testosterone levels (by 50% and 30%, respectively)'.[15]

So, if you vape, please bin it. It's not serving you, your partner or your future child. Once again there is a lot of support out there from the GP, pharmacy, books and apps.

Refined Sugar

If you read 'My Story', you will know this was a tricky one for me. In many ways I felt like I was lying to myself that the sugar did not affect me, as I'm naturally on the slim side, and therefore I could not see the effects in centimetres or love handles. But when I decreased my sugar intake and then got to the point of removing all refined sugar, I noticed the difference in other ways. Those little things in the night no longer woke me up, such as owls hooting, my partner breathing – yes, I said breathing not snoring, that's how much of a light sleeper I was until I did a major detox. Then my energy soared naturally. I no longer needed three coffees a day, my emotions settled and my skin, well, I never again got that one 'period' spot I'd had every cycle since I started my period aged sixteen.

There is mounting evidence to suggest that consuming excessive amounts of refined sugar can indirectly contribute to infertility in various ways, and this is a tricky one to conquer for many people. Even five years in, I stumble too, and this is my job, and I like to think I practise what I preach. I certainly walk the talk.

Excess refined sugar consumption can trigger low-grade inflammation in the body, which can have negative effects on reproductive health. You might not notice the low-grade inflammation until it builds up over years, but then boom: you have developed chronic inflammation. Chronic inflammation can and more often than not does interfere with the normal functioning of the reproductive organs, as it massively disrupts the menstrual cycle and impairs the release of eggs from the ovary, and affects the quality of sperm too. If you are in a couple, at least you can buddy up on giving sugar the shove, as it's easier as a team to stay on track. Look out for areas of inflammation in your body, such as achy joints, gout (a common one in my male clients with low sperm results), redness in the face.

Refined sugar is everywhere. The other day I was in London trying to get food prior to meetings and I popped into a leading high-street supermarket at the railway station. I picked up a packet of pre-packed beetroot and it had sugar in it. Surely beetroot is naturally sweet enough! I popped it back on the shelf. Next, I reached for some fresh turkey slices, and the ingredients listed were turkey, water, salt and brown sugar. I wasn't expecting to find sugar in my meat . . . In the end, I came out with cheese and celery and had them with my homemade gluten-free oat crackers that I never travel without.

Be prepared, folks, just like a Brownie or a Scout.

You will start to realise how careful you need to be, not only when buying food from a supermarket, but also when eating in restaurants. Start to embody attention to detail, and practise the habit of turning over packets when purchasing anything you have not made yourself. Avoid sauces, glazes and marinades on menus or ask the server what the ingredients are in certain dishes. Information is power. Save the sugar for things that you would expect sugar to be in, such as dark chocolate, fruits, honey or cake! Not added to your already naturally sweet beetroot.

Hormonal imbalances: consuming refined sugar can lead to a rapid increase in blood sugar levels, causing a surge in insulin production. Elevated insulin levels can then go on to disrupt the delicate balance of other hormones, such as oestrogen and testosterone, which are crucial for both female and male reproductive health. I'm here to help you protect and balance those hormones! Hormonal imbalance can negatively affect ovulation in women and sperm production in men, potentially leading to infertility. When you do reach for a piece of cake or a chocolate bar, stop and think. Why are you dependent on the sugar? What is the sugar fix masking? Is it stress? Fatigue? Lack of protein? Lack of quality sleep?

By masking the call of your body (yes, your body has a voice. And all too often we gag that voice, because that is how we have socially been trained), you fail to address the root cause of why you are sugar dependent or have a 'sweet tooth'. You don't really have a 'sweet tooth': you are addicted to sugar, and you are deficient in some area or areas of your life that need attention.

Think H.A.L.T.

Ask yourself: Am I Hungry?

Often people are lacking in protein, so they snack on sweet things, or perhaps they have skipped a meal.

Am I Angry?

I for one am an emotional eater, but now, if I feel my emotions rise, I journal, do a meditation, or do a quick box breathing session to slow the adrenaline rush and lower the cortisol levels back down.

Am I Lonely?

A fertility journey can be one of the loneliest times going. Reach out to a friend, have a Zoom call, go for a walk, do something you did as teens, and have a laugh. Life can often get too serious as adults and it's our inner child that is left alone in the playground of life stuffing another cupcake.

Am I Thirsty?

We're often dehydrated. I would say 80% of the clients I work with do not eat enough water. Yes, I said eat, not drink. Many people do not drink enough water either, and those that do often merely flood the body with water and then all they do is pee it out. What you need to be doing is hydrating the body with water foods such as cucumber, lettuces, celery, kale, courgettes, radishes, melon and dark berries, as the body absorbs this kind of water more efficiently on a cellular level. So, eat your water!

Prescription Drugs

Many people are taking prescription drugs such as painkillers, disease-control drugs or antidepressants. I must make this clear: never ever skip, stop or lower your dose of medication unless guided to do so by your medical professional or medical team. I am not a doctor, and you have been prescribed that medicine to help you in your life.

However, you can dig around the internet and see if there are any contradictions with your current medication and fertility fitness, then arm yourself with the data and take it to your medical team and see if there is an alternative drug that will be more fertility-friendly or even whether you can lower the dose. There are always options that will allow you to support your fertility and wellbeing at the same time. This is why I believe in an integrative approach to wellbeing, and that being transparent about your fertility journey with your GP and medical teams is a must. Always be open about supplements too, as they also may have contraindications with prescribed medicines.

Painkillers

While there's still some debate among medical professionals, some studies suggest that ibuprofen might have a negative effect on men's sperm. A group of fourteen young men took the drug ibuprofen at its maximum daily dose for several weeks, and the researchers compared their hormone levels to those of a second group that received a placebo. After fourteen days, the ratio of testosterone to luteinising hormone, which stimulates testosterone production, decreased in men taking ibuprofen.

Also, what are you masking with the painkiller? You are in pain because the body is saying help, so investigate why. There are also many other alternatives to painkillers out there with lots of clinical data to support them, such as high-dose omega-3 for headaches.

The NHS guidance on ibuprofen for fertility is to avoid it.[16]

'This is because taking ibuprofen [tablets, capsules, granules or liquid] in large doses, or for a long time, can affect ovulation. This can make it more difficult for you to get pregnant, but you will usually start ovulating normally again when you stop taking ibuprofen.'

Antidepressants

If you or your partner are taking antidepressants, it's important to be aware of the potential side effects on fertility. While these medications can be incredibly helpful in managing mental health, they may also have some impact on both male and female fertility.

For women, some antidepressants have been found to affect hormone levels, potentially disrupting the menstrual cycle and making it more difficult to conceive. In some cases, they can even decrease the quality and quantity of eggs available for fertilisation.

Men too may experience decreased sperm count and motility when taking certain antidepressants. This can make it more challenging for couples trying to conceive.

It's crucial to have an open and honest conversation with your GP or mental health team if you have concerns about fertility and are considering or currently taking antidepressant medication. They can provide you with the most accurate and personalised information for your situation and support you appropriately in your given circumstances.

Remember, mental health is crucial, and finding the right balance between managing your wellbeing and reproductive goals is key.

We have looked at the body, so now let's look at the mind and heart.

The Mind: Rephrasing Negative Self-Talk

Navigating the fertility process can be challenging to say the least. We need to cultivate a positive outlook and also have a safe space to explore what is going on beneath the veiled 'I'm fine', 'I'm good', and 'I'm OK.'

I truly believe that the body listens to our thoughts, what we say to others and what we say about ourselves. Negativity is like poison; it's better out than in. That is why I want you to go out and buy a small A5 notebook. It can be fancy, plain, cheap or luxurious. Whatever floats your boat and lights up your face – that's the one to choose.

You can get creative and customise it, even make it from scratch from your own paper and bind it. I don't care, just grab it first thing every morning, before your phone, before whoever or whatever shares your bed, the dog, the cat, the kids, study books. If you can, grab it even before your morning wee. When you open it up and see those blank pages, I want you to be the most honest you have ever been with any living soul or higher power. Spill the beans and get it down on the paper.

Many of my clients resist this part of the programme. They say they don't need it, journalling is 'not for them', it's 'not a man thing', it's 'woo-woo', 'I'm not arty', 'I don't have the time' and 'I'm not spiritual.' I'm not asking you to be spiritual, arty or woo-woo. I'm asking you to be a human BEING.

We are so busy doing we don't even know how to BE with ourselves. It's often the hardest thing to do, as we are so very out of practice with this basic human function. Often what we resist or brush aside so vehemently is what we most need. More often than not, I find that the clients who avoid this exercise the most, once they give it a go are the ones who have the biggest emotional breakthrough.

An added bonus is that when couples both engage in this daily activity they begin to connect more, the barriers begin to fall and they see a reduction in tension around fertility. They themselves begin to open up more space for love, they create more fun together and the whole 'guilt' thing gets thrown out of the window when they commit to always showing up to the page daily. When you show up for yourself, it's easier to show up for each other, for family, for friends, at work.

Let your thoughts flow freely, no judgement. As you pour your thoughts onto the pages, something magical begins to happen. You will start to ask yourself questions, see signs you missed and listen to your body more, strengthening the communication pathways with your own mind and body. You'll witness unexpected revelations blossoming like beautiful flowers in a garden you didn't know you had even planted there. You will gain a newfound strength and wisdom not only within yourself but of yourself.

When writing these two to three pages every morning, things will come out that will surprise you and you will start to see patterns of thought emerge and things that you may have pushed down begin to push through and rise. I started the practice of morning pages, or 'free writing', as some call it, nearly twenty years ago when I bought the book *The Artist's Way* by Julia Cameron. It's one of the best supplements and sources of nutrition I have ever committed to on a daily basis. As the founder of my nutrition school, The Institute of Integrated Nutrition, Joshua Rosenthal says in his book *The Power of Primary Food: Tools for Nourishment Beyond the Plate*, 'We must be willing to look not only at the food on our plates, but at the experiences that feed us on a daily basis.'[17]

The morning is not over yet. Yes, you may need to set the alarm clock 20 minutes earlier from now on. More than likely you'll need to pop to the loo by now, but still no looking at your phone or getting into conversations with the dog, cat or with your partner. No, keep putting pen to paper and next write three things you are grateful for now and three things you are grateful for in the future; however, both will be written in the present tense.

For example:

Three things I'm grateful for today:

1. I am grateful for my bed; I love my comfy bed.
2. I am grateful for all the yummy food options in my house (there was a time, when I was sick with lupus, that I was dependent on food parcels from the food bank, so this entry is a regular on my morning gratitude list).
3. I am grateful to have two happy girls in my life.

Three things I'm grateful for in the future:

1. I am grateful to have a publishing deal with Headline (if you are reading this book, this entry came into being!).
2. I am grateful I decided to do the cookbook.
3. I am grateful I can now do the monkey bars in the gym.

Starting the day on a positive note is priceless for the mind and the body, as the two are connected by the vagus nerve, which carries signals back and forth between the two. I see this practice as getting your armour on for the day and removing the emotional plaque of the previous day. Just as we brush our teeth every morning to detoxify from the previous night's sleep and start the day afresh, this practice helps us start the day mentally clean and fresh also.

Remember, this notebook is not merely a collection of words; it is a testament to your resilience, your unwavering spirit, and your capacity to create a beautiful future. Trust in the process, and trust in yourself. Let your hand be your guide, let the words flow and, most importantly, let there be no judgement; this is between you and the page.

Relationships of the heart

Homework for the ladies.

The bath exercise
(You can also do this in the shower, but depending on how flexible you are, it is better in a bath, or you could sit down in the shower.)

From many women and some men, the feedback I get is that they feel they are disconnected from their body.

'I'm angry with it.'

'I don't feel like it's my own any more, it's been taken over by IVF.'

'The doctors control my body now.'

This exercise is one I learnt in body psychotherapy when I trained as a method actor, though we had to do it in a room full of people and not in a bath. I transferred the exercise to the bath because I personally like the feeling of water and its attachment to nature. It's all-encompassing for the body and senses. For me, it creates a feeling of being held and being safe, and I hope it does for you too.

I recommend doing this exercise alone when no one is in the house. Set the room up how it relaxes you best. Candles (non-toxic, obviously), maybe some lyric-free music, some oils or bath salts. I just want you to be warm and relaxed. You go to each part of your body and say thank and I love you, a little like a Ho'oponopono Prayer (a Hawaiian mantra that means 'I'm sorry, please forgive me, thank you, I love you'). In this exercise I want you to say why you are thankful and depending on flexibility, give that area a kiss, or you can kiss your hand and place it on that area. When I was overcoming lupus, I used to do this exercise twice weekly, and at times I would cry because I was letting go of so much anger. Behind all anger is fear and sorrow, and I was replacing it with forgiveness and love. For example, I would say to my legs, 'I'm sorry for being so angry with you and I thank you for carrying me around still, even though I'm slow.' After around a month of doing this, I started to be happy and grateful for the body I had once again, and this was a more solid place for me to grow from.

With my clients, I have a lot of resistance to, or shall I say avoidance of, the bath exercise. Some brush it off, stating that it's normal to feel like this and it doesn't matter, and that they are not going to get anything from it. The ones that resist the most, once I persist, I would say easily have the biggest breakthroughs. They return to our next session declaring that they have had a mindset change, and that they've truly begun to love their body and themselves again. If it's too much now, revisit this exercise in a few weeks. Week 9 would be good, as that's when we will be working on re-investing in yourself and being kind to yourself.

The Letters of Love

> 'All healing is first a healing of the heart.'
> Carl Townsend

Last night I had a session with a client who is already a wonderful mother. She is already fiercely invested in this child she has yet to meet, in being the best mother she can be. By working on her past, working on being present, working on her diet, so she is nourished and not merely fed. Near the end of the session, she cried. It was a cry that had a deafening silence to it, as the depth of her emotional pain was immense. One of those cries where a void is pulled wide open. It was a poignant reminder that love, when it lacks a tangible outlet, can turn into anguish. Hence why I invite you to let it out.

The letter exercises that follow aren't always easy, and I prevaricated about which week to place then in, but I wanted to plant the seed early on in your heart, and so you can revisit it when you feel it's the right time.

You can choose to write all these letters, none of these letters, some of these letters. The choice is yours. Your gut will tell you which letter or letters to explore on your fertility journey.

We often express more love for others than we do for ourselves. We need to give ourselves permission to love ourselves.

Many people prefer to do this exercise outside in nature or in bed or in the bath. Choose somewhere you feel safe.

Letter to you from your future child (both men and women)
Write the letter from your future child to yourself, thanking you for all that you are doing, for taking this book in your hand, for the love that you already give them, for the strength and support, for the food you are eating, for the things you have given up, for the new things you are investing in.

When completed, pop the letter in an envelope and seal it. You can then place it under a plant pot at home and watch the plant grow. You can send it out to sea. You can burn it and scatter the ashes while on your favourite walk, one that one day you will do with your child. The choice is yours. I simply invite you to give yourself the love that you deserve and the permission to experience this, to create tears of joy rather than tears of sadness.

A letter to your past babies (both men and women)
This is for anyone who has experienced a miscarriage or failure of implantation.

This was the hardest letter I've ever had to write. It took me many years to write it, but when I did, I felt a release in my heart, an unclenching of something I had held inside for years.

Take your time. Write a letter of thanks to your babies for all they have taught you on this journey, all that they have unveiled, and thank them for their strength for coming so far and for the DNA that they have passed to you so that they are forever part of you. They will stay forevermore within you ladies, and chaps, your partner is walking around still the mother of your child or children. This DNA will also then pass to your next child.

Letter to your mummy (women only)
(Yes, at the time of writing this at forty-nine and ten months, I still call the woman who brought me into the world my mummy.)

Some clients find this task controversial and often shirk from it. However, the women who embrace the challenge can have immense breakthroughs within themselves, within their family dynamic and also with their fertility journey.

Writing a letter to your mummy is about healing the female lineage. She may have passed, she may have never been a part of your life, you may still have hurdles to get over within your relationship, but it's all part of healing the wounds that our body holds. Please remember, ladies, your eggs began the very important start of their existence in this woman's body.

Being a mother doesn't come with a rulebook, it doesn't mean you get it right all the time, or any time for some people. But you wouldn't be here, book in hand, if it wasn't for your mother.

If there is some kind of disconnect in your female line, after writing this letter, I suggest that you follow it up with a navel massage. Massage your navel with a warming oil, such as organic coconut or sesame oil, and say, 'This female trauma ends with me.'

I ask you to write these letters during these twelve weeks. I repeat: it doesn't have to be now, but at some point, because mental and emotional pain is a poison.

These letters are also a space for men to express their feelings. Many men don't get the opportunity to grieve or to express their connection to their babies of the past or their babies to come because they are expected by society to be strong for their partner. These letters are an opportunity for you chaps to communicate with and express love for your children also.

I hope this brings your past and future children closer to being.

A fertility meditation (for men and women)
I really encourage you to do this fertility meditation, especially you ladies. Before developing this, I used to find an array of fertility meditations online and send each client a choice, so they could find their preferred voice to listen to. However, one particular lady didn't gel with any fertility meditations that I sent her, and then it clicked. Why would she? The guide's voice wasn't HER voice, the one that was the loudest voice of all, the one that woke her in the night, the one she lay awake with in the dark hours, the one that berated her when she saw others getting pregnant so easily. What I needed to do to help this lady was transform HER voice.

So, I ask you to do this because we need to replace YOUR voice with a positive internal dialogue that is bespoke to you, your life, your being and your beat and rhythm. As the lines go from a song in the kids' movie *Vivo*, 'I bounce to the beat of my own drum, I'm a wow in a world full of ho-hum.' Let this meditation be your drum.

Day 1: Take a lined A4 sheet of paper and draw a straight vertical line down the middle. On the left-hand side of the page, write down all the negative things society has told you is gospel about fertility. Write down all the negative things you say to yourself. Go for it, let it all out. Then leave it.

Day 2: (It is important to split this exercise up, as it can be emotionally tiring.) Read each line out loud and then write a positive statement on the right-hand side of the page.

Day 3: While recording yourself, say each positive statement from the right-hand side out loud over and over again until it 'drops' in your body. You will know when this happens, as you will 'feel' it. Finally, say, 'Thank you', 'I love you' and 'You've got this.'

Day 4: Listen to the recording every day, once in the morning and once at night, for a week. After that, listen to it once a day, until it becomes your default voice.

If you're on an IVF journey, you may want to do the whole

exercise for each phase of the cycle. So, pre-egg retrieval, post-transfer and then the two-week wait.

Here is an example:

Left side:

    I can't get pregnant.

    I feel useless as a woman/man.

    I can't deal with stress.

    I have high anxiety.

    Everyone but me can get pregnant.

    This is punishment, I must have done something wrong.

    I'm too fat/thin.

    I'm too old.

    I got married too late.

    My eggs are old.

    I'm a failure as a wife/partner/husband.

    I'm letting everyone down.

    I hate my period.

Right side:

My body has the ability to do more than my mind knows.

My fertility does not define me as a woman/man.

I will commit to supporting my stress.

I can lower my anxiety.

I don't know everyone else's fertility journey.

I am a good person.

I will treat my body with love and kindness.

I choose to rejuvenate and not deteriorate.

I waited for the best co-parent for my child.

I still have eggs.

I am doing this because I care.

Committing to me is committing to others.

My period means I am still releasing eggs.

The whole recording should be around 5–6 minutes. You can jazz it up with music intros, white noise, birds tweeting, rain, waves or whatever you feel is most impactful and makes you smile on the inside.

> 'Exploring emotional blockers was a big thing for me. Imagining our future baby, holding on to hope and having this work helped me continue to hold on to hope and, for us, resulted in a beautiful baby daughter after three years of trying to conceive.'
>
> Kat

Week 3. Cleaning Up the Fertility Past

Trigger warning: This chapter mentions abortions and childhood trauma

I struggled with where to place this section in the book, because it's something I normally weave in and out of with clients. I only do it with the client's permission and then only with the client taking the lead. It's dependent on where they are within themselves, their individual fertility journey and, most importantly, their fertility past.

Some wounds in life are still very raw. Please do not see this section as one you must work through if anything discussed does not apply to you. If you read this section and it is applicable to you, please take time to digest it and maybe even give yourself permission to skip over the exercises and revisit them later. At least I have planted a seed in your mind, and maybe it's something you will go on to explore later with a professional. Some of this may resonate with you, some of it may not. So, pick and choose what will serve you and your needs and, most importantly, what you are currently comfortable exploring.

If anything in this chapter triggers you, please ask for help. Asking for help is the biggest gift to yourself and a sign of great strength. Most GPs are great at pointing you in the right direction for all mental health matters or referring you to another professional. I have also listed below some dedicated services in this area.

Free services such as:

The Miscarriage Association: 01924 200799

Pregnancy Crisis Helpline: 0800 368 9296

Doula UK: Here you can find excellently trained miscarriage doulas and postnatal birth doulas (www.doula.org.uk/contact)

I want to address past abortions.

If either you or your partner have had an abortion, this may be a controversial read, but it's something that does come up with my clients, both women and men, and I feel I would be doing a disservice to you if I did not address it or give reference to those who have had to make this decision in their life.

For some people, not all, there is a feeling of guilt that may never have been dealt with, or which wasn't there at the time but has suddenly come into being now there is a struggle to conceive a child. I have been asked a number of times by my clients who have had past abortions, 'Am I being punished for what I chose to do in my teens/twenties/thirties, now that I'm not able to have this child?'

The answer, of course, is 'No'. 'No' this is not some kind of crazy karma or punishment. That was the path that you were on then, and now you are walking another.

Once again, please do ask for help and guidance if this is something you are struggling with, no matter how many years have passed. Because, yes, time can be a great healer for some, but not for all.

There is one particularly helpful exercise I have done with both male and female clients who have had an abortion or abortions in the past. This may be some help to you too, but only if you feel comfortable doing it.

Do not try this if you feel triggered. If you do feel triggered, see this as a sign that it's time to get some professional guidance. Please do not hesitate to reach out to one of the above helplines.

This letter is very similar to the letters that you may have explored, attempted or written last week. This time I invite you to take a walk outside in nature, find a park, a wood, or any place where you are surrounded by nature. Take a pen and pad and write a few words to the child that wasn't brought into this world. Thank them for all they have given you. Thank them for the love they have created within you. For how their coming into being, but not into birth, may have protected you, changed the course of your life. It can be in any format you desire. A letter, a poem, a song. If you are not great with words and you are better with music, create a melody on the guitar or piano or paint a picture. Simply give love and thanks. Let things flow; this is about release and connection. Anything that stagnates is not good for us.

Don't forget about microchimerism too. For those of you who are not into the spiritual side or what some may call the woo-woo bits, this scientific research has shown that the cells from the foetus cross over into the mother's body and can be found in the mother decades later. I hope you find not just peace, but a connective love in this exercise. It's not easy at the start for many, but afterwards there can be acceptance knowing that those cells walk with you each day.

A walk in the park
I've had a number of male clients over the years, a few women also but mainly men, who won't take the supplements I've suggested. There is a block. They don't invest in the rainbow

diet (more on this later), they even continue drinking alcohol or don't attempt to give up vaping. These actions reveal to me that something is preventing them from doing all that they can to realise their dream of becoming a parent, because they do still long for that, even if their partner sees their inaction as meaning the opposite. So, I try to find the root cause, their WHY.

When I get them in a session on their own and we break it down, the same WHY comes up time and time again: they have a fear of becoming a parent. Even though they want it badly, their fear overrides their actions. More often than not, they are worried they will not be good enough or they will repeat the parenting patterns of their parents and continue the cycle of some degree of childhood trauma. Perhaps as a child they felt neglected, hurt or lost within or excluded from the family dynamic. And now, as a grown adult, they are still so very protective of this little child that they don't want to repeat their parents' behaviour, and they fear they will not be a good enough dad.

So, if this is you and you were that child, and a constellation of past events are drumming up some hesitation towards becoming a parent, and it's getting in the way of you investing in your fertility journey, try out this exercise. Or work with a professional to help you unpack and reframe these thoughts.

First take a shower or a bath so you're relaxed and warm. Then I want you to lie down or sit somewhere comfortable and prepare by doing a few rounds of box breathing or a 10-minute guided meditation. Next, with your eyes closed, I want you to visualise a safe space in nature. It could be somewhere you feel warm, like on a beach or a walk in the woods wrapped up in your favourite coat and woolly hat. It could be a park, a field, a wood, a lake. It doesn't even have to be a place that you've been to. It could be a place you have longed to visit, somewhere you have seen in a movie or that you keep as a screen saver. It doesn't even have to be real; it can be a made-up place from your dreams. Wherever it is, I want it to fill your senses: touch, smell, sight and taste. When you are in a place of wonder, even the air tastes different, and it's that magical place I want you to visit in your mind.

Walk around this beautiful place you have chosen and immerse yourself in nature's perfect symphony. When all your sensory cups are full and the weight and tension of the day has dropped from your shoulders, I want you to look around and find an inviting place to sit. When seated, take your imaginary shoes off if you're wearing them and place your bare feet on the ground. Feel the earth beneath your feet and a warm light going through your soles to the central core of the earth. Take a deep breath then let out a huge sigh. Visualise a child, a cute-looking kid (yes, it's you), playing not so far away from you.

Simply observe them and watch them play for a while. Then I want you to connect, make eye contact and smile. If they do not smile right back, it's OK. Offer to play with them. You break their perhaps cautious mood by revealing you are a safe space, by being open and letting them feel and know you are all love and softness. Then invite them to sit on your knee and give them a huge hug, one of those hugs that no one, no matter how hardened they are, can help but surrender to.

Look down at them, enveloped in your arms, and say, 'I love you, you are safe, you are important.' Once the child smiles back and snuggles in, I want you to tell them a story. You open your magical book.

The book is the story of YOU. All the wonderful things that are going to happen to this little child of wonder. How they found friends who loved them just the way they are and how they fell in love with romantic partners and were loved back. How they travelled, ate different foods, laughed till they cried. Anything and everything: it's your story, not mine.

Keep going and watch how the child reacts. I want you to wait until the little you starts to smile, and then the smile turns into a laugh and the look of wonder grows in their eyes. They settle in your lap and snuggle in closer, and the closer they get to you, the deeper into the story they will be.

You will get to a point where you turn the page and the pages become blank, as this is the story so far. Now you offer them a set of coloured crayons, and the two of you start to draw a colourful picture together. When the picture is complete, I want you to stand up and offer your hand. Once they accept your hand, I want big you and little you to walk hand in hand towards the right of the frame and then directly out of frame. This little child is no longer scared and lonely; they now have you, wonderful, mindful, proactive, kind and loving adult you.

They are no longer a scared little child on their own, they've walked into the wonderful world of now.

Past Births

When I started my fertility journey the last time around (in my forties, already with a grown teen and two births under my belt), I found that most of the fertility books out there spoke to the reader as if they'd never had a child before. That this child-in-waiting would be the reader's first pregnancy and birth. Which may not be the case for many of you reading this book; you may have already given birth, and you may have unresolved issues and fears around that or those births. Those past births could be fuelling your anxiety around your current fertility journey.

These feelings are not exclusive to the female either. It's not uncommon when I'm working with a couple for the man to feel anxious because he has seen his partner struggle, perhaps physically, emotionally or both. They could have experienced a traumatic birth last time. Their partner may have struggled emotionally and physically with the hormone fluctuations of pregnancy. And now they fear going into another round as they don't want their partner to take the burden and potentially suffer once more.

Or it may be the birthing parent who has reservations about the delivery, because last time they needed clinical intervention for the birth to happen and that trauma has not been unpacked. So here I encourage you to not only talk to each other, but talk to a friend or someone who is trained in such matters as this, like a birth trauma postnatal doula. It doesn't have to be a recent birth for you to do a little work on it, especially if it's casting a shadow over this fertility journey. I have had clients who have seen a birth trauma postnatal doula fifteen years postpartum.

As we now know, trauma, especially unresolved trauma, can affect the body's physiology, and turn on the stress response. This in turn can create imbalances in hormonal responses. It also affects us emotionally and can create a divide within a couple. So I do recommend that, if this is something that needs unpacking for you, you connect with someone to facilitate the healing process.

As I mentioned at the start of this chapter, I wasn't sure whether to include this section in the book. But just like that, I got a sign. I can't quite believe how the universe works. As I'm typing away, literally at this point, an old client sent me a message and photograph of her seven-month-old baby. 'Thank you so much for suggesting the trauma counselling,' she wrote. She truly believed it helped her conceive the little bundle of joy in the photo. Her first experience of childbirth had been so traumatic that she had almost blocked it out. She and her baby had nearly died. During her pregnancy she'd had terrible hyperemesis (where you suffer from intractable vomiting, leading to weight loss and volume depletion throughout), and as a result of all this she had PTSD that was making her body shut down. Once she understood that and dealt with the trauma that she and her baby had experienced, and the amount she had suffered both mentally and physically in the pregnancy with her counsellor, she got pregnant. I know this isn't a magic wand for everyone, but you may relate to her experience, or it may shed a little light on something deep inside.

Dealing with birth trauma can be overwhelming and isolating, even between partners, as we often don't voice our feelings because we don't want to overshadow others' emotions that are being or have been expressed.

For example, I had a miscarriage at twenty weeks in my mid-twenties, and it was something that I felt I needed to clear before going into my third birthing experience. Out of all my pregnancies, that loss was the longest labour in terms of time, the most physically painful, the one that I lost the most blood from and the one where I had to stay in hospital the longest.

I live in England, and quite often we Brits suffer from a stiff upper lip. A cup of tea, a cry, some flowers and chocolates are meant to heal all. Traumatic events are packed up and stored away deep inside and sealed with a smile that makes others say, 'Isn't she coping well?' We're often commended for being stoic after a miscarriage, while we're going through IVF or after a traumatic birth experience. Maybe it's helpful for some. But my stoic smile was a mask; my experience left a lot of physical and emotional scars around pregnancy and birth.

I waited some twenty years to speak to a birth trauma doula about my experience. It was only when I was on my fertility journey at forty-three that I felt I could no longer carry the weight of it into the pregnancy that I so wished for. Speaking with a birth trauma doula was one of the best things I have ever done for myself. It was a couple of hours with a wonderful lady, a couple of hours I wish I would have gifted myself many years before, if only I'd known such a person existed.

Our past often weaves in and out of our present; only once we know or admit to what is there are we able to choose what will serve us to take into the future. I hope this chapter allows you to understand that there is a place for this, there is a place for you to share, for you or your partner. It's not just the ladies, after all, as men can hold on to traumatic events too, and we all need a safe space to talk and work through them. Once we can voice it, it is then we can truly begin to heal.

Week 4. Supplements

I'm sure a lot of you will skip forward to this week. What you'll find here are the foundations of fertility support. You will also find more in Week 11, The New Kids on the Block; these newbies are the ones you most likely won't find in other books.

If you have picked up this book or you're listening to my Northern lady voice on audio, it is more than likely you are already taking some kind of fertility supplement, most likely a fertility multivitamin. If you have the bottle or packet to hand, please pop the book down and see what's in it. For now, ignore all the jazz and clever marketing on the front and look at ALL the ingredients listed on the back. Is it loaded with fillers and bulking agents and even artificial sweeteners?

Not all additives are inherently problematic. In fact, some can serve important functional purposes. Some additives can actually help improve the absorption and bioavailability of the key nutrients in the supplement. This ensures your body can effectively utilise the beneficial vitamins, minerals and other compounds. Additionally, some ingredients may be added to ensure consistency and accuracy in the dosage from one capsule to the next. This guarantees you get the intended amount of each ingredient per serving.

However, it is best to find a supplement that is produced by a brand that prides itself on being free of bulking agents, or at least does not include any of the below ingredients. Some products even have these ingredients featured multiple times in their ingredients.

Think of these as the DIRTY FIVE (that won't make you thrive):

1. Titanium dioxide: Used in many supplements in the UK and USA. This white compound is commonly used to make capsules appear brighter, but studies have raised concerns about its potential to damage DNA (think of the effect this could have on your egg and sperm quality; remember, DNA fragmentation is often cited as a male infertility factor). France banned sales of food products containing titanium dioxide (E171) in 2020.
2. Magnesium stearate: This is used as a flow agent to help powders move through manufacturing equipment.

However, it doesn't actually deliver magnesium to the body and may be linked to autoimmune issues. Also, it's not one of the eleven types of magnesium that you are looking for to help stress, cramps and sleep. Actually, if you ingest too much magnesium stearate it can have a laxative effect. This is due to it irritating the mucosal lining of your bowels, causing your bowels to spasm and triggering bowel movements or diarrhoea.

3. Palm oil and hydrogenated fats: These are often used as lubricants, but excessive consumption is associated with increased 'bad' LDL cholesterol and cardiovascular risks.
4. Talc: The European Union banned the use of talc as a food additive in 2010. Enough said.
5. Maltodextrin: Maltodextrin may disrupt gut flora by promoting the growth of certain bacteria while inhibiting beneficial ones, potentially leading to digestive issues and a compromised gut barrier. We are all aware now that we need a happy gut; a happy gut supports a happy mind. Additionally, it's important to note the high glycemic index (GI) of maltodextrin. The GI of maltodextrin is typically in the range of 85–105, which is considered very high.

To put this into context, the glycaemic index of table sugar (sucrose) is around 65. So, as a health coach, I think it is important to make you aware that this might show up regularly in your supplements.

To show you how common these ingredients are, these are the first few ingredients in the no. 1 brand of fertility supplements in the UK:

Maltodextrin, Bulking Agent: Microcrystalline Cellulose, Vitamin C (Ascorbic Acid), Magnesium Oxide, Inositol, N-Acetyl Cysteine, Tablet Coating (Hydroxypropylmethylcellulose, Polydextrose, Talc, Medium Chain Triglycerides, Glycerin, Colours [Calcium Carbonate, Iron Oxides]), Ferrous Fumarate.

I also want to emphasise that just taking supplements is not and never will be the answer. There are so many contributing factors when it comes to health and wellbeing. You can eat all the kale in the world, juice, do smoothies, go paleo, keto, or whatever you want your diet to be for longevity, religious or ethical purposes. But if you're stressed out due to your personal demands of life, work, family, finances, you have a leaky gut, you pile toxic chemicals on your face and body, you cook in toxic pans and then clean your fertility-boosting salad bowl using a toxic dishwasher tablet, your body is going to be having a hard time absorbing the nutrients from your supplements. It will also have a high demand for nutrients that your supplements may not be meeting, and it's going to have a hard time detoxing.

This is why food is first. Always. (We will be covering food in Week 8. I wanted you to really look at your lifestyle first, though, to understand how this is maybe contributing to deficiencies.) But I do believe that supplements have a place, especially with fertility. This is because the quality of our food has decreased, as well as the fact that we live in such a fast-paced world. Why have I placed the supplement section weeks before the food section? Because it may take weeks for you to get your blood work taken and then wait to get your results. It could also take a while for you to source which are the purer brands that are filler-free. Some brands have very clear transparency and give you access to their independent testing online. I have listed some in the trusted sources section at the back of the book.

In the wellness world, at times I do get flak for encouraging the use of supplements, as food should conquer all, apparently. Yes, it should. But unfortunately, as you will see, it doesn't always cut the mustard, and we then need a little help from pills and potions. Also, I would note that different periods in our lives require different support; fertility, pregnancy, postpartum, perimenopause and menopause will all need different levels of support in the forms of food and supplements for the body and mind.

This is why below I list all the basic supplements individually, along with the amount that has been clinically proven to aid fertility. Many multi-fertility supplements only contain a nominal amount of these ingredients rather than the amount that has been clinically tested to make any kind of a difference. Many brands further confuse the issue by showing the amount included in the supplement alongside the daily recommended amount. However, the daily recommended amount is for people who are not trying to conceive. This is not to be confused with a daily recommended amount for those who are trying to conceive, however. This is not always made clear to consumers and is misleading.

There are a few smaller supplement brands on the market who, in my opinion, make great fertility supplements for females and males; however, I would say there is a wider choice out there for the ladies. But even these brands sometimes exclude important nutrients like magnesium, as to get the correct amount of magnesium into the capsule along with all the other ingredients would make it too big to swallow daily comfortably. Or they know certain nutrients, such as vitamin C, will be more available within food than others. So, just be aware that not everything is necessarily covered.

A note before we go ahead. I'm not a fan of 'throw the kitchen sink at it and hope for the best'. What I lay before you are a number of supplements that have been studied and proven to enhance fertility. However, always remember you are an individual and thus you need to supplement according to your bioindividuality. You need to look at your diet, blood work and stress levels to see what you might need. These are things you need to bring up with your GP, gynaecologist, urologist and at your first IVF appointment. Just because a friend took something and they got pregnant, it doesn't mean it's right for you. You must always be transparent with your medical team, because they can only treat you to the best of their knowledge with all you present them.

The supplements I most recommend are:

Women

B vitamins
Omega-3
Vitamin C
Choline
L-arginine
Pycnogenol
Coenzyme Q10
Folate
Shatavari
Vitamin D
Myo-inositol
Probiotic

Men

Zinc
Vitamin C
Omega-3
L-citrulline
Ashwagandha
Pycnogenol
Coenzyme Q10
Folate
Vitamin D
Vitamin E
Selenium
Probiotic

Omega-3

Healthy fat is fuel for the egg and sperm. Think cute, chubby baby!

One study states that 'In infertile women, omega-3 fatty acid intake has been associated with increased probability of pregnancy following IVF.'[18] This does not mean it does not improve natural fertility, simply that there is conflicting evidence regarding proof in this area due to the lack of controlled studies. Obviously, it's easier to have a controlled study within the confines of IVF.

> 'Absence of proof is not proof of absence.'
> The Reverend William Wright

Omega-3 fatty acids, particularly those high in eicosapentaenoic acid (EPA), play a crucial role in fertility. These essential fats are not only vital for overall health (especially mental health) but have been specifically linked to reproductive wellness. I think it's also vital to use supplements to support your mental health while on this journey, as it can certainly be taxing on the mind. Plus, while you are protecting the brain, you are protecting the gut – the good old gut–brain axis.

EPA-rich omega-3s are renowned for their anti-inflammatory properties, which help reduce oxidative stress and maintain optimal cellular function. Remember that high inflammation is often a contributing factor to failure of implantation.

I'm a Cancerian and I often jokingly put my star sign down as the reason behind the fact that I love fish and seafood; I could eat it every day from breakfast to supper. However, I live with a family who have other ideas when it comes to fish, so incorporating fish into my meal planning can be tricky. Plus, good-quality fish can be rather costly. Only yesterday I went to the local fishmongers and got a tiny pot of crayfish, two very thin fillets of smoked trout, tiny slithers almost, and a fillet of trout, and it came to the grand total of £16.45. This covered my breakfast and lunch on Saturday and will make my dinner on Sunday for one, as my family are away. However, I can get a whole organic chicken for £17 that will feed my family of three for at least three evening meals (different recipes), two adult lunches and be the base of a soup that will cover four adult meals. I know I'm not comparing the nutrition content, but both are good sources of protein, yet one is totally out of my price range to have on a regular basis.

Add another layer to the mix. The actual omega-3 content of the fish itself.

According to a 2016 article in *Scientific Reports*, ' . . . a single 130g portion of Scottish salmon farmed in 2006 would have been adequate to meet the 3.5g EPA+DHA weekly intake level set by ISSFAL [the International Society for the Study of Fatty Acids and Lipids], whereas in 2015 this would have required two portions.'[19]

Add to the fact that the general guidelines for consumption of EPA and DHA are based on data that is decades old. The way of life for most of the population has changed as well as the food sources and the food quality, so I think we need to bear this in mind when we think about how our diet might cover the available sources of nutrients that we need to support fertility.

A 2016 study on omega-3 levels in farmed salmon stated, 'If the current trend of decreasing levels of EPA, DHA, vitamin D and micronutrients in farmed salmon continues, we may well need to eat more fish to provide similar health benefits than those described previously. Future recommendations for fish intake, which are currently based on cohort studies that were performed one to two decades ago, when EPA and DHA intake from fish was probably significantly higher than it is now, will need to take account of this.'[20]

So how much should you be aiming for?

When it comes to omega-3 fatty acids, there isn't a specific recommended daily amount that's been officially established, and it's also different from country to country. But most health organisations suggest that healthy adults should aim for 250–500mg of omega-3s per day. But that's healthy people.

That said, when trying to conceive, whether through natural means or with the help of fertility treatments, many doctors and fertility specialists actually recommend a much higher dosage – over 2,000mg of omega-3s daily.

Also, how do you know where you already are? What levels of omega-3 do you currently have in your body? It wasn't until I was a couple of years into my fertility coaching that I found out you can do at-home testing for omega-3 levels. If you can, I think it's important to know where you are starting from, as we all have individual needs. The trouble with most healthcare systems is that we are all treated the same. One OBGYN from the USA I interviewed called it the 'cookie-cutter system'. This is also true when it comes to supplements. This is why I favour single supplements, as it is more tailored to bio-individuality and not a blanket formulation for everyone. For example, you may already have a higher level of vitamin D in your body but low levels of omega-3, so why should you take the same fertility multivitamin as someone with low vitamin D levels and higher omega-3?

At-home tests in the UK cost around £35.

I like at-home testing not only because of its convenience, but because then, after three to four months, you can test again and see if the supplementation is doing its job. We may not notice an external or internal change, but that doesn't mean it's not happening. Also, if you are taking a multivitamin, it's difficult to test and see what is actually making the difference. Plus, if you are not absorbing a vitamin or mineral, that could be an indicator of something that needs further testing and investigation by your health practitioner. But if you don't have the levels to show them, they won't know.

Omega-3 and men

Think: Fish will help your swimmers!

Omega-3 fatty acids, particularly DHA, are widely recognised for their importance in supporting male fertility. The benefits that omega-3s have on the enhancement of sperm motility, allowing the sperm to swim more effectively towards the egg, is a great low-cost way to get your swimmers closer to the golden egg. Long-term supplementation, longer than three months, has also been seen to increase sperm concentration and optimise sperm morphology, ensuring the sperm are healthy in both number and structure. Additionally, and this is, for me, the most powerful part, omega-3s protect the DNA integrity of the sperm, preventing the fragmentation that all too often impairs fertilisation and embryo development.

A study published in 2024 found positive results from the use of omega-3 supplementation. 'Supplementation with omega-3 fatty acid results in improvement of sperm concentration and total motile sperm count in infertile men with oligozoospermia.'[21] The study supplemented with 1g of omega-3. Note that that is double the maximum daily recommended amount. (Now do you see why I say be careful of being swayed by percentages on a fertility supplement label?)

A supplement may only contain 250mg of omega-3 and can legally state it contains 100% of your daily recommended amount of omega-3. However, this is not only the lower end of the recommended daily amount, but also only a quarter of what has been used as a benchmark in human studies and had positive results in altering the sperm profile!

There is a mountain of clinical evidence in human studies that supplementation of omega-3 is vital to those struggling, especially with unexplained infertility. Hence why I strongly encourage both men and women to source a good-quality omega-3 with a high concentration of EPA and DHA.

When taking an omega-3 supplement, you will be able to get a higher concentration when it's in liquid form. However, it's not to everyone's taste and it also may not be practical due to work and travel, as it will have to be refrigerated. So, look for good-quality capsules that have transparency and also sourcing on their website, so you know you are getting good-quality, naturally sourced omega-3.

Vitamin D

With many of us working indoors, be that at home or in an office, factory, school or shop, and our main source of vitamin D coming from sunlight, most of us are not getting enough vitamin D. Other factors that affect vitamin D absorption from the sun include the colour of our skin and body fat.

When I was researching for this book how much time the average person stays inside, it truly shocked me. Even I (as a health coach, who should know better) spend the majority of my day inside, especially so while writing this book. What follows may encourage you to get your vitamin D levels tested and maybe explore a vitamin D supplement, but also to take breaks outside throughout the day, no matter how cold it is. I, for one, will try to take a long walk on my lunch breaks. We have shunned sunlight somewhat over the years, with the increase in awareness of skin cancer. But we need it to stimulate and reset the body.

The latest IPA TouchPoints research found that the average time spent inside the home is now 18 hours and 43 minutes per day, compared to 17 hours and 37 minutes per day in pre-lockdown 2020. The 'indoor generation' refers to the growing number of people who spend the vast majority of their time indoors. This has become increasingly common in recent years due to modern conveniences, working from home, and technological advancements such as the internet, smartphones and video games.

A 2018 study by YouGov asked 16,000 members of the public in fourteen countries across North America and Europe about their perceptions of indoor living. It found we believe we spend 18% of our time inside (so about 4 hours). In reality, it's closer to 90% (about 21 hours).

In October 2021, the British Nutrition Foundation commissioned The National Diet and Nutrition Survey, which found that almost 1 in 5 adults in the UK have low levels of vitamin D in their blood and that 49% of adults are unaware of UK Government guidelines for vitamin D.[22] Observational data suggest a link between low 25-hydroxyvitamin D (25-OHD) levels – the best measure of Vitamin D status in humans – and an increased risk of adverse pregnancy outcomes, such as gestational diabetes, pre-eclampsia, infections, Caesarean section, and foetal growth restriction.[23]

Wow fact: Several studies and reviews have highlighted the potential role of vitamin D for female fertility. 'Interestingly, in northern countries, there is a seasonal variation in pregnancy rates, with a peak in summer and autumn, i.e. the seasons with the highest serum 25(OH)D concentrations.'[24]

According to Anne Merewood, an assistant paediatrics professor at Boston University School of Medicine, vitamin D-deficient pregnant women are nearly four times more likely to end up having a C-section.[25]

So why is vitamin D important for fertility?

Vitamin D plays a vital role in regulating hormone levels in the body, including testosterone and oestrogen. And we know we have to have those in balance to create not only a healthy libido but a healthy reproductive system. Vitamin D also enhances your mood and, as a fertility journey can be a stressful time, you need your mood to be as calm as possible. When you are stressed, have anxiety, or low mood, your libido is going to plummet.

Optimum levels of vitamin D have been associated with improved blood flow throughout the body. This is something that I talk about a lot, and you will see that blood flow is vital for good fertility, which is why a lot of people turn to acupuncture.

Vitamin D is also something you can get tested at home or by your GP (if they are open to such tests – some are, some are not).

An at-home test in the UK can cost from as little as £4.

Who may be at risk of low vitamin D levels?

The importance of checking vitamin D levels for women who are overweight or with darker skin is a no-brainer as far as I am concerned, as they are at a higher risk of vitamin D deficiency. Vitamin D is particularly crucial for women with certain reproductive health conditions, such as polycystic ovarian syndrome (PCOS) or endometriosis. Note, the NHS is in firm agreement on the importance of vitamin D, but in my opinion their suggested range is too low.

Women who have experienced recurrent miscarriages are more likely to have a successful pregnancy if they have enough vitamin D, so please get tested. Some women I have asked to get tested are in the low 20s. One lady's vitamin D level came in at 13nmol/L. Her GP had previously thought she was depressed. When the doctor prescribed her high-dose vitamin D, both her mental health and her reproductive health vastly improved.

Another lady had chronic fatigue, her libido had vanished, and she was using sugar to boost her energy. No one had tested her vitamin D levels, even though she is Pakistani British-born, worked crazy hours as an accountant and had the added pressure of studying for more exams. At our initial meeting for a taster session, I encouraged her to get her vitamin D levels checked, and when she got her results, they were so low that she was able to take them to a clinic and get an IV of vitamin D to raise her levels to within a safe range. At the time of writing, she is now 32 weeks pregnant naturally, in her forties, and all scans show that the baby is healthy.

Furthermore, a study in 2022 found that a vitamin D

deficiency could increase your risk of miscarriage by 94% and increase your risk of recurrent miscarriage by 4 times. It also found that vitamin D deficiency in the male partner was also a contributing risk factor.[26]

How much do you need?

Anecdotally, 75% of my clients (female and male) find out after testing they are deficient in vitamin D by NHS standards.

The NHS says that the 'normal' range is anything above 50nmol/L.

The WMA (the World Medical Association) gives a different recommendation.

'Vitamin D has [a] major role in calcium and bone metabolism. Normal values are 75–100 nmol/L (30–40 ng/ml). Vitamin D deficiency is defined if serum hydroxyvitamin D levels are less than 50nmol/L (20ng/ml), insufficiency as 50–75nmol/L (20–30ng/ml).'

Many fertility IVF clinics around the world recommend that the ideal concentration is between 50–100nmol/L. With this in mind, I would want you to aim for around 75nmol/L.

This is why I encourage all my clients to get blood work done by the GP first before they even do their first session with me. You also never want to overdo it with any supplement, especially vitamin D. It's about establishing balance.

Folic Acid or Folate – the Great Debate

Folic acid historically is the first pill we ladies think to pop for fertility prep. But pause a moment and let's delve a little deeper, because there has been much debate over the last few years over the best form.

Many people opt for folate over folic acid nowadays. Folate is the natural active form of the vitamin that is more readily absorbed and utilised by the human body. It's the form your body recognises. Folic acid is the synthetic form, and your body will need to convert it first to make it bioavailable. So, if you use the synthetic form, your body needs to work harder unnecessarily. Additionally, some individuals have a gene variation that affects their ability to efficiently convert folic acid, making folate a more suitable option. This is the MTFHR gene, and you can have a mutation of this gene that means your body is unable to efficiently convert synthetic folic acid into its active form, 5-methylenetetrahydrofolate (5-MTHFR). You can get tested for this, and I believe, where fertility is concerned, it's worth doing so.

With this in mind, I would encourage you to look for the natural, active forms of folate, such as 5-methyltetrahydrofolate, folinic acid or methylfolate when choosing a supplement, as these are more readily available for the body's needs.

Recommended daily amount of folate for women (NHS and the CDC): 400mcg from before you're pregnant (ideally three months before) until you're twelve weeks pregnant. At this point, your antenatal team may increase the dose.

Folate for men too!

The recommended amount for men is also 400mcg, but, surprisingly, folate is not common in many male fertility supplements. And yet some studies show that levels even as high as 700mcg can have a positive effect on sperm.

A 2021 study states: 'Folate deficiency has been shown to increase DNA strand breaks.' They conclude that 'supplementation with zinc and folate can have noticeable effects on semen quality and these may improve natural fertility and success rates with fertility treatment.'[27]

A 2020 systematic review and meta-analysis showed evidence of associations between paternal folate status and sperm quality, fertility, congenital malformations and placental weight.[28]

This is great news for men. If you are in a couple, you can bulk buy this supplement and save some money.

Vitamin C: The 'C'arrier Vitamin

Vitamin C is often referred to as a 'helper' or 'carrier' vitamin because it plays a crucial role in facilitating the absorption and utilisation of other essential nutrients in the body.

One example of this is the way vitamin C interacts with glutathione, a powerful antioxidant (glutathione is featured in Week 11, The New Kids on the Block). Vitamin C helps to recycle and regenerate glutathione, ensuring the body has an adequate supply of this important compound.

Similarly, vitamin C enhances the absorption and activity of vitamin E, which is yet again another essential antioxidant. Vitamin E is fat-soluble, meaning it requires a carrier molecule to be transported and utilised effectively in the body. Vitamin C helps here as the carrier and it also helps to convert vitamin E into its active form, allowing it to be more readily available for the body's needs.

A quick note here to recommend that you steer away from the effervescent fizzy tablets that are popular, as they are often full of fillers. Food first, then a simple powder will suffice. You can get 500g ascorbic acid (vitamin C) for £15 – that's just under a year's worth right there.

Vitamin E

Vitamin E is great for both sexes, but especially men. It plays a crucial role in supporting male fertility by protecting sperm cells from oxidative damage. Low levels of vitamin E can lead to decreased sperm quality and motility. Motility is especially important for those going for natural conception or IUI, as low motility will make it harder for sperm to reach and most importantly fertilise the egg. Additionally, vitamin E's antioxidant properties help maintain the integrity of sperm DNA and protect against damage. This is something to bear in mind because DNA fragmentation can often be a significant contributing factor in the failure of your embryo to make the transfer stage in IVF and lead to early miscarriage.

Vitamin C/Vitamin E male combo

A 2005 study showed that the combination of vitamins C and E can significantly reduce DNA damage in sperm. The amount given in the study was 1g of vitamin C and 1g of vitamin E daily for 2 months.[29]

Collagen

Collagen is not just great for your skin or for menopausal ladies like me, but it's also super beneficial for fertility too. It's another fairly low-cost supplement that can be easily included in your daily life. You can add it to your morning coffee or to smoothies. I have even popped it in soups, homemade bread and muffins, and no one has been able to tell. It's also one of the few supplements that more often than not comes in powder form rather than capsule, and therefore it's less likely there will be fillers in it. If there are, bin it.

Collagen can benefit both female and male fertility, so you can bulk buy to get a cheaper deal. The production of collagen naturally begins to decline around the mid-twenties for both men and women, and this decline accelerates with age. For women, the decrease in collagen can impact the health and elasticity of the uterus, as well as the quality of the eggs, leading to potential fertility challenges. It also supports the development and maturation of ovarian follicles, which contain the eggs, and may help improve egg quality.

Collagen and men

Collagen declines at a rate of 1% per year after the age of thirty, so if you are a forty-plus male reading this, your collagen has vastly declined. In men, the decline in collagen can affect the structure and function of the testes, prostate and seminal vesicles, potentially resulting in reduced sperm quality and overall male fertility. Research suggests that collagen supplementation may help improve sperm quality and overall male fertility, but it's not something that has been heavily researched at present. However, just because the researchers are not investing in studies, doesn't mean you don't have to consider collagen as an option.

Collagen can be obtained through dietary sources, such as bone broth, meat, fish and dairy products. However, for individuals who may have difficulty meeting their collagen needs through diet alone (like me, as I don't eat red meat and I'm not a major consumer of dairy, bar Parmesan and the odd bit of feta), a collagen supplement may be a beneficial option to explore. Plus, you can get it in all forms that support ethical dietary and religious choices. Bovine, marine and plant-derived collagen are now widely available. I must say that some of the marine options do smell of rotten fish, so I tend to go for bovine or plant-derived. I feel they mix better into my coffee too, and don't alter the taste of my drinks.

Once again, look for a company that has transparency about their sourcing. This is another reason why I favour bovine collagen, as I can source it from organic or outdoor-bred animals. Some areas of the sea have their own issues with mass pollution and heavy metals such as mercury. I don't want these in my supplement, and you shouldn't either. So, look for companies that show levels of mercury especially, as well as independent third-party laboratory testing on their product.

L-glutamine

L-glutamine is not something you see in most female fertility supplements, which in my humble opinion is bonkers, because it's an amino acid that is a powerhouse when it comes to fertility.

Not only does it improve your egg quality but your gut health too – a double win, seeing as research suggests links between gut issues and recurrent pregnancy loss.[30]

This is another supplement that often comes as a tasteless powder, so it's easy to mix into smoothies and cold drinks.

Ashwagandha
(often called Indian ginseng)

I love the multicultural world we live in and how ancient medicinal practices such as Ayurveda and Traditional Chinese Medicine are now so easily accessed by many. One common

Ayurvedic herb is ashwagandha. It's a plant that has been used in Ayurvedic medicine for over 6,000 years. Many people take it for stress, anxiety or sleep.

However, it's not for everyone, and when taken should be cycled, i.e. two weeks on and then a week off. Always remember that one person's medicine can be another person's poison. What I mean by this is not everything is for everyone. That's the whole point of this book – we are bio-individual. This is why I often prefer single-ingredient supplements, as you can skip ones that may not be supporting you.

Please note that people with thyroid issues or autoimmune conditions, anyone taking anxiety medication and anyone who has a stomach ulcer should avoid this herb.

For those who can take ashwagandha, it can be great for fertility, and it is especially beneficial and transformative for MEN. Yes, chaps, I have your back!

Numerous studies have demonstrated the positive influence of ashwagandha on sperm motility, which you know by now is a crucial factor in natural fertility.

One study found that ashwagandha supplementation significantly improved sperm motility in infertile men. The researchers reported a 57% increase in sperm motility in the ashwagandha group compared to the placebo group.[31]

Another study, published in 2013, examined the effects of ashwagandha on semen quality in infertile men. Twenty-one men in the treatment group received 225mg of encapsulated ashwagandha root by mouth 3 times daily for 12 weeks. The results were outstanding. 'When comparing semen parameters at baseline and after the 90-day treatment phase, average sperm concentration rose corresponding to a 167% increase in sperm concentration in men treated with Ashwagandha root.' There was a 53% increase in semen volume in men and a 57% increase in sperm motility.[32]

These statistics could be life-changing – or life-forming – and this is a natural herb that is relatively inexpensive.

A review article analysed the available evidence on ashwagandha's impact on male reproductive function. The authors concluded that ashwagandha was effective in enhancing sperm motility, in addition to increasing testosterone levels and improving overall semen quality.[33]

The mechanisms by which ashwagandha improves sperm motility are not fully understood, but it is believed to involve its adaptogenic properties and ability to reduce oxidative stress. Ashwagandha may help optimise the hormonal environment and support the overall health and function of the male reproductive system, leading to enhanced sperm motility.

Shatavari

Shatavari is a wonderful herb and one I have used many times personally. I feel it grounds me, and it has been a wonderful support during a number of stressful times in my life. It's great for hormones, and, for me, my hormones are the first thing to go astray when I hit a wobbly time. It also has a very feminine fertile meaning. The name 'shatavari' is derived from the Sanskrit words *shat*, which means '100', and *vri*, which means 'root'. The word *vari* can also mean 'husband', which therefore translates to 'she who has a hundred husbands'. So, it promises a lot and, more often than not, it delivers. It's great for ladies with PCOS and follicular growth development issues, as it nourishes your ovaries. Many studies have shown that it's great for your libido too – double whammy.

Note to ladies with fibroids: This herb has been shown to worsen fibroids, so skip this one.

For the chaps

Shatavari is going to regulate your hormones too. I guess, until now, you gents most likely haven't thought much about your hormones, but I'm making it my mission that you not only think about them but you also start to invest in them.

Several studies have found that shatavari supplementation can improve sperm parameters in men with fertility issues, including increased sperm count, motility and morphology, so that's pretty much everything. It comes in pill, capsule or powder form, therefore it's easy to incorporate into your daily routine.

Note: Avoid shatavari if you are allergic to asparagus.

L-arginine

Women after the age of thirty-five may want to add 1–2g of L-arginine if your protein intake is low, as this can be a game-changer when it comes to fertility. Whether you're aiming for natural conception or going through the IVF process, this supplement can give your fertility a boost because it improves blood flow. Remember, blood flow is pivotal to the implantation stage because it improves the lining of the uterus, creating a more nurturing environment for the implantation process.

In men, L-arginine has been found to improve sperm production, motility and morphology. By increasing the blood flow to the testicles, it aids in the production of healthier and more active sperm.

L-citrulline

You may not be familiar with this one. L-citrulline is an amino acid made by the body. It converts to L-arginine, which boosts nitric oxide production. Nitric oxide helps your arteries relax and work better, which improves blood flow throughout your body. L-citrulline and L-arginine are essential components for the body to produce nitric oxide. While L-arginine needs to undergo a complex breakdown process to be effectively used, L-citrulline directly boosts intracellular levels of L-arginine, increasing nitric oxide levels more efficiently than just taking L-arginine on its own.

One study demonstrated that a higher intake of L-citrulline, especially when combined with pycnogenol, resulted in significant improvements across all semen parameters. This highlights the potential benefits of supplementing with L-arginine and pycnogenol for enhancing male reproductive health. Once again, it's all about blood flow, which is why practices like acupuncture aid both male and female fertility.

General rule for men is to take 2g of L-citrulline daily.

Tongkat ali

Tongkat ali literally means 'Ali's walking stick', which refers to its aphrodisiac effects. Yet another gift from nature. This one is more for you chaps.

One of the ways tongkat ali has been shown to support sperm is by improving sperm morphology, which is often one of the common low factors for men. Tongkat ali's ability to boost testosterone levels may contribute to improved sperm morphology results, as testosterone plays a crucial role in sperm development and maturation. It also has properties that may help reduce inflammation in the male reproductive system, which can otherwise negatively impact sperm quality and morphology.

Melatonin

Melatonin is a hormone produced by the pineal gland in your brain that plays a role in sleep. However, it's not just for sleep; it's also found in high levels in the ovaries and follicular fluid.

This one is for the ladies. You cannot legally get it over the counter in the UK, so you will need your fertility doctor to prescribe it if they think you are a good fit for it. Please do not get it randomly from the internet, especially if you're doing IVF, as you need to take it at a certain time and a decided amount under the guidance of your medical team.

There is a lot of very complex data out there on this topic. Many studies show inconclusive data, but this is often due to how the study was conducted. There are studies that show great results with better-quality embryos and higher rates of implantation in women undergoing IVF treatment. However, further extensive studies are essential to explore the specific effects of melatonin on aspects such as miscarriage rates, live birth rates and overall pregnancy outcomes. But it is definitely one to discuss with your fertility team from the offset.

Zinc

Listen closely, men. Numerous studies have indicated that zinc supplementation can enhance sperm motility especially and overall volume and morphology, particularly in sub-fertile men. This is a vital trace mineral that many of us are not getting enough of. In fact, it is worth nothing that around 17% of the global population is affected by zinc deficiency. Given zinc's critical role in sperm development, it is logical to assume that higher zinc levels can have a positive impact on sperm quality.

However, enhancing sperm quality with a zinc supplement, as with ANY of the supplements suggested, is not a universal solution, as various factors come into play. How old are you? What's your diet plan like? Are you vegetarian? Do you smoke? (Hopefully not by now, but if you do, you will more than likely have low levels of most vitamins and minerals, so this is something to bear in mind.) With that said, most studies suggest that consuming 30mg of zinc daily can greatly improve sperm quality.

Selenium

Another vital trace mineral that plays a crucial role in sperm health. It acts as an antioxidant, protecting sperm cells from oxidative stress, which can damage DNA and reduce motility. Selenium helps regenerate and recycle glutathione (glutathione is featured in Week 11, The New Kids on the Block), ensuring it remains active in fighting off free radicals and other harmful substances. In essence, selenium supports the antioxidant properties of glutathione, contributing to overall cellular health and immune function. It's great for your thyroid, mood and cholesterol, as well as low cost.

Clinical data suggests 100–150mcg daily improves sperm. However, you could save some money on your supplements and eat some Brazil nuts instead (if no one in the home has a nut allergy). Just one Brazil nut contains 96mcg of selenium. I know I'm talking about diet here, but not everyone can or does eat nuts.

Probiotics

Unless you have been living under a rock lately, you will be aware that gut health is key to all health, and fertility is not excluded from that. The reproductive system does not act in isolation.

DHEA

DHEA is a hormone whose job it is to help produce other hormones; therefore, it is called a 'pro-hormone'.

DHEA is naturally produced in various parts of the body, including the brain, ovaries/testicles, and the adrenal glands. It plays a vital role in the production of both oestrogen and testosterone. Levels peak in early adulthood and, like many things, declines as we age.

Research suggests that supplementing with DHEA could enhance pregnancy rates for women with low ovarian reserve. Several studies have shown promising results, including increased pregnancy rates and improvements in follicle counts and egg retrieval during IVF cycles.

The positive effects observed were mainly in women with diminished ovarian reserve, and DHEA has not been proven to help those with normal ovarian function or increase egg counts for women undergoing egg freezing procedures. DHEA supplementation is not for those ladies with a history of sex hormone-sensitive cancers, such as breast, ovarian or endometrial, and it can also have a negative impact on those with PCOS. With this in mind, only take DHEA if it is prescribed by a doctor who is familiar with your fertility circumstances, as they will know if it is a good fit for you, when to introduce it and for how long.

Maca

Maca is a wonderful earthy plant that grows natively in the high Andes of Peru and Bolivia. I love maca and personally take it daily because it's a powerhouse of essential minerals, vitamins and antioxidants, boasting impressive levels of key nutrients vital for overall health. A typical 10g serving will supply you with 4.5mg of calcium, which surpasses the calcium content found in milk, so it's great for vegetarians or those who do not tolerate dairy. Additionally, maca provides 20mcg of selenium, 9.9mg of arginine and 7.6mcg of riboflavin (B2), all of which are listed in this section as supporting fertility.

Black or red maca for men

Studies suggest that maca may help improve sperm, especially quality, count and motility. This adaptogenic herb is believed to support hormonal balance, including testosterone levels, which is essential for male fertility.

Red maca for women

This adaptogen is renowned for its ability to help balance hormones and regulate menstrual cycles. It can also boost women's libido. When choosing maca for female fertility, it is recommended to opt for gelatinised maca powder. Gelatinisation is a process that removes the starch content from the maca root, making it easier to digest and absorb. You can get it in powder or capsule form. Personally, I use capsules, but the powder can be easily added to smoothies, etc.

Progesterone

Ladies, if you are 'catching', as I call it (having a chemical pregnancy or miscarrying very early on), the possible use of progesterone is something to bring up with your fertility team.

Progesterone is frequently recommended for women with low levels of this hormone, those experiencing irregular menstrual cycles, bleeding in early pregnancy, and those who are miscarrying early on.

This hormone is essential for preparing the lining of the uterus for the implantation of a fertilised egg and for sustaining a healthy pregnancy.

Back in 2021, The National Institute for Health and Care Excellence (NICE) published updated guidance on miscarriage, stating that women at a high risk of pregnancy loss should be offered the hormone progesterone. NICE recommends progesterone to lower the risk of miscarriage in women who experience bleeding in early pregnancy and those who have experienced at least one miscarriage.[34]

The guidance also states that progesterone may not prevent every miscarriage and that more research should be conducted in this area. But yet again, if this is you, it's important to discuss whether this is suitable for you with your doctor.

Choline

This is one I didn't know about, even while studying and during my initial training. I found out about choline when talking to a number of obstetricians and gynaecologists at the start of my fertility coaching. Many of them were frustrated that it is not something as commonly considered as, say, folate when it comes to fertility, and it really should be.

Choline is an essential nutrient that plays a vital part in fertility; it's particularly important for the production and maturation of both eggs and sperm. Unfortunately, it's not in a lot of prenatal supplements and, if it is, it's not in the amount that has been shown to make a difference. So, once again, read the labels and look at the smaller brands that are more conscious about having the correct amounts and not deceiving people who are often struggling to meet their child.

Choline is a precursor to the neurotransmitter acetylcholine, which is involved in hormonal regulation and signalling within the reproductive system. Inadequate choline intake in women has been linked to increased risk of infertility, miscarriage and birth defects. In men, choline deficiency can impair sperm quality, motility and overall reproductive function.

Choline vs folate

Choline is often confused with or overlooked in favour of folate, but they are not interchangeable. Both choline and folate are crucial for reproductive health, but they have distinct functions. Folate is primarily responsible for the proper development of the foetal neural tube, while choline plays a more direct role in the health and function of the reproductive organs and gametes (eggs and sperm). So, they are both crucial.

Iron

Iron is crucial for female fertility, as it plays a vital role in the production of healthy eggs and supports a regular menstrual cycle. Iron deficiency can lead to anaemia, which may disrupt ovulation and overall reproductive health. Iron also supports the transport of oxygen to the reproductive organs, promoting a healthy environment for implantation and a smoother pregnancy.

I'd suggest you check your iron levels every three to six months and go over your blood work results with your GP or fertility team.

B Vitamins

Vitamins B1, B2, B3, B6 and B12 are essential for various metabolic processes in the body, including energy production, hormone regulation and overall reproductive health, so a B complex can be helpful.

Vitamin B12, in particular, has been highlighted for its importance in female fertility. For women who are undergoing IVF, sufficient intake of vitamin B12 has been shown to enhance the effectiveness of this process and increase the likelihood of a successful pregnancy. I'd suggest getting your B12 levels regularly checked every 3–4 months.

PQQ (pyrroloquinoline quinone)

PQQ is a unique compound that is beginning to get more of a spotlight when it comes to female fertility and egg quality. I have to admit, I only stumbled upon PQQ when researching this book. As a powerful antioxidant, it helps protect eggs from the damaging effects of oxidative stress, and there have been significant human studies showing its positive effects on IVF results.

Myo-inositol

Myo-inositol is not just beneficial for women with polycystic ovarian syndrome (PCOS), it can also be advantageous for all women, especially those over the age of thirty-five who are on a fertility journey, including those undergoing IVF.

Myo-inositol is essential for the growth and maturation of oocytes, as it aids in regulating the signalling pathways that influence these processes, ultimately resulting in the production of higher-quality eggs. Research indicates that supplementing with myo-inositol can lead to improved IVF outcomes, especially regarding embryo quality, implantation success and pregnancy rates.

Additionally, myo-inositol has been linked to a reduced risk of chromosomal abnormalities in developing embryos.

There are some contraindications with myo-inositol, as it may affect certain medications, including lithium, antidepressants and blood thinners. Also note that since myo-inositol is primarily processed by the kidneys and liver, individuals with existing kidney or liver diseases should either avoid or limit the use of myo-inositol supplements.

I know it's a lot to navigate, but it is important to understand what is what when it comes to fertility supplements. It's also important to know which will be helpful for YOU, which is why I always suggest getting blood work done and looking at your diet and lifestyle to home in on what needs extra support.

> 'It was really refreshing to have Liberty highlight the issues that can arise with male fertility in a world that often focuses on female fertility as a primary issue when struggling to conceive. With her guidance, we increased my sperm count threefold through simple dietary and lifestyle changes and now have a beautiful sixteen-month-old daughter.'
>
> Harry

Week 5. The Four Pillars of Health

In the Western world, fertility fitness is often approached in the same way that many medical professionals approach any type of health obstacle – by 'fitting the pill to the ill'. Don't get me wrong, I love a supplement and often suggest them to my clients. I take them myself daily. However, if you don't prioritise the foundations of health, in essence you're throwing your money down the drain when you invest in supplements and good-quality food. Because without the foundations, you are not giving the 'investments' the best chance. You won't get the best bang for your buck, as the body has to fight hard just to carry out its basic functions. Instead, we want to focus on the fundamentals before the repair work can even begin. My four pillars of health that I like to work on with my clients are mostly free or very low-cost. They are SLEEP, HYDRATION, BREATH and MOVEMENT. We are focusing on just three here because one is so significant it deserves an entire week of its own – sleep. I've found that sleep hygiene and establishing a sleep routine have been major challenges for my clients, so I've set aside Week 6 specifically for this topic.

Hydration

Hydration is key to female and male fertility.

Think of it as basic maths. If 83% of your blood is water and we need good blood flow for fertility, then it becomes a no-brainer. I ask my fertility clients to consume two litres of water a day as a minimum. No matter your height or weight.

However, this is the benchmark for those NOT exercising, and you should be exercising. So, you also need to replace the moisture that you're losing during exercise. Keeping hydrated is important for nourishing the fluid around your fallopian tubes and the fluid levels in the endometrium as it prepares to look after your foetus. Hydration is especially important for the ladies taking drugs for IVF, and especially those who are taking steroids.

You chaps don't get out of it either. To support optimal sperm health, it's crucial for men to stay properly hydrated. Without sufficient water intake, sperm quality can suffer, leading to a decrease in volume and concentration. In fact, water plays a vital role in supporting the fluidity of sperm. Moreover, dehydration can hinder the body's natural detoxification processes, which are essential for reducing the toxic burden and ultimately boosting sperm count and sperm quality.

As a guide, I would suggest two litres of water a day minimum. Eat at least two watery foods for lunch and dinner and then listen to your body. Like I say, the body knows best. So when you go for a wee, have a look at the colour, and when you go for a poo, have a look too – is it dry?

Urine key

Pale yellow wee or clear wee means you're doing well.

A dark yellow or amber or even brown wee means you need to start flushing out the toxins with some good water.

Yes, I did say 'good water'. I will expand on this in Week 7.

Do you EAT enough water? And, yes, you read that correctly, you need to eat your water.

I personally drink around two to three litres of water a day. But I ALSO focus on watery foods, especially now my skin is changing due to being perimenopausal.

Prime ways to eat your water:

90–99% water content: cantaloupe, strawberries, watermelon, lettuce, cabbage, celery, spinach, pickles, squash (cooked)

80–89% water content: apples, grapes, oranges, carrots, broccoli (cooked), pears, pineapple

If your skin is drier due to age and a dip in hormones, or your poo is drier due to your cycle, which can happen around the luteal phase (after ovulation and before menstruation) when progesterone levels peak, make sure you eat a couple of these for at least two of your meals each day.

EAT AND DRINK your water to detox and keep hydrated every day.

So much in the fertility world is a big expense, but this one is easy and readily available.

Breath

Time and time again when I speak to clients, their breath seems to be stuck in their chest, and when they talk, the rhythm is staccato. In the modern-day world, we often lead very fast-paced lives, and we have become fast-paced shallow breathers. We dance the paso doble when we would benefit from the stretched-out notes of a waltz.

I invite you to take a big, deep breath in and hold it. Did your shoulders go up to meet your ears? Did you suck your belly in? Did you strain your face? Now I want you to close your eyes and imagine your baby is already here and you are staring in wonderment at how phenomenal their existence is, watching the rise and fall of their belly. When babies breathe in, their belly balloons, and when they breathe out, their belly deflates. At some point in our lives since the time when we were babies, we've all forgotten how to breathe properly.

Research has shown that the way we breathe can influence our fertility, with both men and women being affected. The key lies in the balance between our sympathetic and parasympathetic nervous systems. When we breathe incorrectly, our sympathetic nervous system, also known as our 'fight or flight' response, is triggered. The sympathetic nervous system is responsible for a lot of chaos in our bodies, and can lead to stress, anxiety and hormonal imbalances. This can negatively impact fertility, making it more challenging to conceive.

When we breathe correctly, more nasally and into the belly first rather than shallow chest breathing, our parasympathetic nervous system, responsible for relaxation and calmness, is activated, promoting a more fertile environment. The problem is that many of us breathe in a way that is opposite to our natural design. Over the next few days, make a conscious effort to breathe correctly first thing in the morning, check in a few more times during the day, and then again before sleep. This will help you to get out of sympathetic mode, which is not 'sympathetic' in the normal sense of the word to the fertility process at all.

Movement

Too little or too much movement can affect your fertility; as with everything, it's about balance.

Working out what movement supported my fertility was a biggie for me when trying to conceive in my forties. Before my fertility journey, I religiously made it to the gym at the end of my road five days a week for a minimum of an hour, but I also topped this up with classes. Additionally, I had a personal trainer once a week, which was hardcore, plus I trained twice a week in stick fighting. After suffering with lupus, I knew how movement supported not only my body but also my mental heath, and the truth be told, it was this one thing I was reluctant to change when it came to my fertility. I knew that I was more than likely placing a lot of stress on my body, but I never thought about my menstrual cycle and how my body was under different natural stresses at certain times of my cycle. Yet think about how women are different to men and how we run on a different cycle to men throughout the month. So, this begs the question: should we train the same as men?

The way I was training with such intense and prolonged physical activity had the potential to disrupt my hormonal balance and not support the fertility path I was on.

So I started to train according to where I was in my cycle.

Here is a guide to exercising and moving to support your menstrual cycle. It's about supporting the body by working with its natural rhythms and getting the most out of your exercise.

The bleed: menstruation: days 1–7: opt for gentle, low-impact exercises like walking, flow yoga or swimming to help reduce cramps and promote a sense of calm due to the loss of blood.

The follicular phase: days 7–13: invest in your high-intensity workouts like strength training, spin classes, stick fighting (if that's your bag too).

The ovulation phase: approximately day 14 (not everyone is the same): this is when we get a peak of testosterone, so let's use it! Get boxing, run, HIIT, do circuits, book your PT in.

The luteal phase: days 20–23: focus on relaxation techniques like stretching, resistance bands, physio work, flow yoga, jogging, swimming, and up your breathwork with some Kundalini yoga to help manage premenstrual mood swings.

The late luteal phase: days 24–28: low resistance, long walks, swimming, flow yoga and Pilates.

On the other hand, if you are a couch potato, get moving, as a lack of physical activity can lead to obesity, insulin resistance, and other metabolic issues that can contribute to an unexplained infertility diagnosis. Research suggests that moderate exercise, such as brisk walking, cycling or swimming, can actually improve fertility in both men and women by boosting overall health and increasing the quality of sperm and eggs. This is about creating a way of being that supports your fertility and your longevity. The fitter you are now, especially if you are a woman, the more likely it is that you will have an easier pregnancy and a smoother delivery. So find what that sweet spot is for you when it comes to movement for the body and the mind.

If you find movement overwhelming, don't rush to join the gym or force yourself to do an hour a day. Little and often helps.

Top tips:

1. Use the stairs, not the lift.
2. Walk up the escalator.

3. Park your car 10 minutes' walk away from the station.
4. Where possible, implement a couple of walking meetings at work.
5. If working from home, schedule in 10-minute breaks for star jumps, laps around the garden, etc.
6. In the lighter evenings, go for a walk after dinner.
7. If you already have little ones, when they are in bed do 15 minutes of yoga or Pilates.
8. Buddy up – we are more likely to move if we have a friend to do it with. You can even do it on Zoom.

I had a client who simply added in 20 minutes of movement to her day six days a week and she lost a stone in a month. Be the tortoise not the hare and it will become part of who you are, rather than feel like a fad or a chore.

Week 6. Sleep

Why did I give this pillar of health its own chapter? Because out of the four pillars of health, sleep is generally the one that's all over the place for my clients. It's also the one that has taken me years to master, but now I guard my sleep as fiercely as a lioness guards her cubs.

If you already have little ones or are a shift worker, take from this chapter/week what you can. Perhaps try practising Yoga Nidra to recover from a dysregulated sleep pattern. As I know, having the opportunity to sleep or plan to sleep may not be open to all, but when it is, please do invest in yourself.

I always have a conversation with my clients about sleep within the first few weeks of working with them, and more often than not it goes like this:

Me: 'What time did you go to bed on Saturday night?'

Liberty Mills

Client: 'One o'clock, maybe two, probably three by the time I fell asleep. I'm not sure, I just know it was late.'

Me [asking again, this time in a slower voice]: 'What time did you go to bed on Saturday night?'

Client: 'Two thirty in bed.'

I'll then ask them a third time, sometimes even a fourth.

Me: 'You're intelligent. I know you are. Think about what I am asking, literally. What time did you go to bed last night? And remember there is power in language.' I emphasise the word *night*.

I see the penny drop.

Client: 'Oh, I didn't. I went to bed Sunday morning.'

Me: 'So, you didn't go to bed Saturday night at all, you went to bed the same day you woke up?'

Client: 'YES.'

I believe that nature knows best. We mostly follow the rhythm of the sun, rising when the sun rises and going to bed when the sun has set. We adjust our clocks, watches and phones to the daylight cycle. Most people (excluding shift workers) work during the day and sleep at night.

The majority of people stick to this pattern during the week, but when the weekend arrives, instead of going to bed at 10pm, for example, we stay up late partying or watching TV, often going to bed at 2am – because it's Friday night, because it's Saturday night. Regularly disrupting our sleep patterns like this can have a detrimental impact, especially on a woman's menstrual cycle. Think about how, when you travel long-haul, a woman's menstrual cycle can go out of sync – whether it's a delayed period or a bleed that's different from the norm.

Now imagine you've stayed up later on a Saturday night. See, even I did it – I said 'night' instead of Sunday morning. If you pull an all-nighter (for me an all-nighter is missing the crucial part of sleep between 10pm and midnight and going to bed the next day, even if it's pre-dawn). You feel awful until Tuesday, at which point you vow to 'catch up' with an early night. By Thursday, you feel burned out and depleted from work and modern-day stress, so you binge-watch a boxset to 'treat' yourself and start the cycle all over again. Essentially, for your body, it's like jumping between time zones without the perks – no suntan, no beautiful beaches, no one making your bed in the morning – and you still have to turn up to work and bring your A-game.

Work isn't the place to sleep off the effects of travel-style disruptions. You can't lounge on a sunbed with ocean waves in the background, an unread book on your lap, and a cocktail by your side – unless you have a particularly sassy job!

You can't really cheat sleep either. While practices like yoga nidra or NSDR (non-sleep deep rest) may help compensate somewhat, the way most people cope with a lack of sleep is by relying on stimulants: caffeine, cigarettes, sugar and scrolling on social media (yes, that dopamine hit feels good, but it comes with an almighty crash).

Many people tell me, 'I can survive on five hours' sleep.' I don't doubt that for one minute. But I don't want you to just 'survive'. Sooner or later, missing sleep catches up with you. It's called burnout. I've been there – with lupus – and let me tell you, it's not pretty. No more surviving. I want people to thrive.

And we need your body to thrive – not just for your future health but also for your reproductive health and wellbeing. We don't want tired-out eggs or stressed-out sperm. We need to respect and honour the brain's sleep-wake system, which regulates melatonin and cortisol levels – key messengers to other hormones. When we are deprived of adequate sleep, both in quantity and quality, the body produces more stress hormones. This isn't just harmful to overall health; it can disrupt oestrogen, testosterone and other reproductive hormone levels. Clinical research suggests that the body's internal clock, the circadian rhythm, is linked to reproductive hormones that stimulate ovulation in women and influence sperm maturation in men. Sleep is one of the best ways to protect your body – and it is free!

If you don't have a regular sleep pattern, you are directly interfering with this delicate and precise process. This can contribute to menstrual irregularities in women, making it challenging to predict ovulation, which is a crucial part of planning conception. A lot of my clients are stressed-out business women who are working till ten or eleven o'clock at night, and some even get up in the night to work for an hour or so on a deadline or a project and then go back to bed.

These women all have one thing in common: their ovulation is not regular and so it's harder for them to 'organise' sex at the 'the right time'. Plus, when you work crazy hours, you are often too fatigued to have sex or you may not even be in the same space to have sex. As a couple you may also have come to an arrangement and decided that the late worker will sleep in a different room. This can create a huge disconnect in relationships, and you are also missing out on spontaneous opportunities for sex if this is your lifestyle pattern.

It's not just the ladies, it's men too. Poor sleep quality can result in unhealthy sperm, reducing the chances of successful fertilisation and increasing the risk of complications or unviable embryos; therefore, it could be a contributing factor in failure of implantation in natural conception.

Ladies, take heed: lack of sleep can seriously affect your hormones. If the above did not shift your mindset, maybe the science will. Many studies show the effects of poor sleep on fertility.

A 2015 study states: 'High levels of thyroid-stimulating hormone (TSH), as seen in hypothyroidism, can cause anovulation, recurrent miscarriages, amenorrhea and menstrual irregularities. TSH appears to increase prior to sleep onset, and continues to increase over the course of the sleep period/night, and then decreases during the day. Under acute sleep deprivation TSH surges, whereas under extended sleep deprivation, TSH may become diminished.

'Oestradiol is secreted by the granulosa cells in the ovarian follicles and regulates FSH and LH, playing a critical role in ovulation. When oestrogen does not rise and fall appropriately, FSH and LH may not be able to stimulate ovulation ... Women with regular sleep schedules had 60% lower levels of oestradiol than women with more variability. High levels of oestradiol were also related to poorer sleep quality.'[35]

Remember how I said at the start of the book that you are my client? With my clients, sleep hygiene is non-negotiable.

Sleep Hygiene

It's common for people to prepare in life, whether for birthdays, weddings, weekend activities or sports; for example, most people would not dream of signing up for a marathon and not preparing for it. When you arrive at the gym you do your warm-up with stretches, followed by gentle cardio, to support not only the efficiency of the workout, but to protect your body from injury. But when people get to one of the most important factors of human existence, fertility, they fail to prepare with some of the most basic practices, especially the most fundamental one of all . . . sleep. Modern life does everything in its power to sabotage us getting to and staying asleep, with TV, phones and stimulants such as sugar and alcohol galore. It seems that sleep is just something that must be done, rather than a time that is cherished.

As a new parent at the age of twenty-three, I knew from all the books on child rearing I devoured from the library (I had never even held a baby, so I decided I should get all the advice I could get from experts in the field) that it was important for my child's health and development to train her into a good sleep pattern. Children thrive off this routine, and then they become ballsy teenagers and think they know best and rebel and throw it all out of the window. It's only when the body says 'NO', when we burn out or get sick, that we revisit what our parents so carefully curated for us as a child.

So, how can we prepare for sleep?

Let's look at my five-year-old as an example. A non-negotiable is her wind-down time before bed. This is a good hour or so where there is no TV, no overstimulation. We do some crafts, colouring or some gentle play (often I have to tell her daddy it's *gentle* play and so no goblins growling, no running around like dinosaurs or putting evil witches upside down in the cauldron).

What wind-down time looks like:

When upstairs, she may have a bath, and I'll massage her with a children's magnesium lotion or she will simply rub it on her own feet, as, in her own words, it helps her 'dream of rainbows'. This will be followed by me or Daddy or both of us reading her a book or two with the lights low. If she is not ready for sleep when we leave after cuddles and kisses, she will get a book out herself and attempt to follow the story from the pictures, and sound out the odd word, by the light of her reindeer light. She intuitively knows that this is what slows her down. She doesn't get her Kindle out and load up *Dragon Rider*.

On the rare occasion that we abandon this routine, at Christmas for example, and she's watched a brightly coloured fast-paced movie later than normal, followed by running up and down her grandparents' house with her cousins and, let's be honest, a lot of sugar too, it's very difficult to get her to sleep. By the time we do get her into bed, she says she is not tired, or sleep is boring, or she wants TV. She is literally a nightmare to calm down to a point where she is ready for sleep. After a night like this, the next day she is also thrown off course. She doesn't want cuddles in bed (our normal wake-up routine), she is grumpy and demands TV and snacks. She doesn't want her usual fruit porridge and a glass of water and a chat at the kitchen table. Instead she will throw a tantrum and demand chocolate or crackers and she'll want to eat in front of the TV. Her body and brain want those stimulants again for the dopamine rush.

Adults are no different; think back to the last time you had a late night. The morning after, you were likely more inclined to opt for a chocolate croissant or a smoothie with banana and honey and a coffee for breakfast over a protein and veggie option. You may have had a scroll on social media before you even pulled back the duvet. We are still so very similar to toddlers. But I believe we need to listen to our body's needs over our mind's wants. I invite you, for the next two weeks, to parent the toddler in you. Remember, there will be tantrums, so if you are in a couple, parent each other. Start to create a bedtime routine that is non-negotiable.

Sleep prep: Ninety before Nightie

'Ninety before nightie' is 90 minutes of wind-down time before you go to bed.

I will use myself as an example. I have an alarm that goes off at 8.30pm to remind me it's wind-down time. This signals to me that it's time to tell everyone (mainly my mummy and my eldest daughter, who has a family of her own) that I'm switching off all digital forms of communication for the evening and I'll be back online the next morning.

For you this could be time to finish up those last two emails.

Tell your loved ones you'll be in at home from this time onwards in case of an emergency.

Don't worry, I'm not going to make you go cold turkey. The first week, turn your phone off (yes, I would also like you to have no TV or Kindle – basically no devices). And I mean off, not silent, 30 minutes before you enter the bedroom. The week after, turn it off 45 minutes before you enter the bedroom. The week after, make it an hour, then an hour fifteen. In a month you'll have reached the full hour and a half.

Not only does this stop you being hyperstimulated before bed, it also gives you free time for some of the exercises we have already looked at and some of the exercises that will be coming, such as navel massage, fertility meditations, self-love meditations, journalling and gratitude lists. You can include other activities, such as an evening walk after dinner, or even talking to your partner. You could include some non-sexual intimate time too by giving yourself or your partner a massage, or just play some cards or read one of those many books you've been meaning to read but have never got around to. I don't really care what you do, as long as it relaxes you and relaxes the brain and doesn't involve a screen.

I said turn off your phone before going into the bedroom. I would prefer it if there were no mobile phones in the bedroom at all. If it's a must, then place them near the door or at the end of the bed and make sure they're on airplane mode. If you need to be contacted in an emergency – maybe you have family living all over the world, older parents, grandparents, or your partner works away – go old school and get a house phone with a cord (remember those? You may not, but they worked perfectly well back in the day). The great thing about the house phone was that it came with unspoken universal boundaries. No one sent you a WhatsApp message at 11pm, Amazon didn't notify you at 5.30am that your parcel had been dispatched, your favourite clothing line didn't message you that it was launching its discount sale at midnight.

When you have a house phone, ONLY give the number to your nearest and dearest, then you know that if the phone rings in the middle of the night that it *is* an emergency. With a house phone, you can safely WhatsApp at 9pm 'Good night, I love you' and then turn your phone off. They can reach you if they need to.

Also, purchase an alarm clock so you don't need the phone anywhere near your bedroom. I say this because, even if the phone is at the end of the bed or just outside the door, some people are so addicted that they just can't help themselves, they need one last fix. But thankfully I have also found that if the phone is on the other side of the closed door, along a corridor, down a flight of stairs and on the other side of another closed door, many people can't be bothered to have one last check of celebrity gossip, one last rant on X or a final scroll on Instagram or TikTok. When you remove the phone, you prevent what potentially is not just a quick scroll but an epic trip into another time zone.

The alarm clock not only saves us in the evening, but also in the morning, as how we start our day is so important in regards to how the rest of the day plays out. If we have our phone lying on our bedside table on airplane mode, we still have to turn the alarm off and then the device is in our hands. And once in your eager hands, the body turns on the sense memory and the brain knows all too well by now that it will deliver the inevitable dopamine rush. We tell ourselves all kinds of stories, 'I'll just check the weather', cue glee, or 'Boo, let's just stay under the covers for another five minutes.' Or 'I'll just check my bank balance', cue glee if it's payday or gloom if a direct debit you forgot about has taken you overdrawn. Then there's, 'Oh, I'll just check if Jane texted me back about Pilates on Saturday.' Or 'I'll just catch up on a few emails while I'm in bed on my phone.' And on and on.

Step away, step away, step away, to keep deregulation at bay.

This kind of morning behaviour immediately puts the body into fight or flight. This means you are already starting the day off on the back foot and this is before you've even had a glass of water or a wee.

The final thing I want you to buy is a watch. I used my phone to tell me the time until a few years ago and was surprised at the amount of screen time I was clocking up. I decided to get a watch instead, one that only told the time. Please, no watches that ping you emails or ones that tell you what your pulse rate is and how many steps you've done. I mean a good old-fashioned tick-tock watch that has hands. I state this because quite often we look at our phone to check the time as we're going about our day. We jump out of the shower. How much longer do I have? I just finished my makeup. How much longer do I have? I'm having breakfast. How much longer do I have? Then we get sucked into checking emails, notifications, WhatsApp, LinkedIn, when we were only checking the time.

How much is your screen time?

Get your phone out. I bet it's close by, or you may even be reading this on your phone . . . Look at your settings and see where your screen time is divided up. It can be very enlightening and insightful to see where we are investing our time and, seeing as time is one of the things that most of us say we don't have enough of, here is an opportunity to gift yourself some back. Set a time limit of how long you will be on socials. Or if you are like me and you work on social media, you can get an app that blocks you out of certain apps after a certain amount of time. I have found this immensely helpful.

Weighted blankets (the hug blanket)

I have a history of not being a great sleeper since adulthood, and it is even worse when sleeping away from home. That is, until I stayed at my best friend's house and tried her weighted blanket. I was flat out for nine hours. I had not slept for nine hours since I was a teenager, unless I was sick.

The science behind weighted blankets lies in the concept of deep pressure stimulation, which mimics the gentle, soothing pressure of a hug. Research has found that we need four hugs a day for survival, eight hugs a day for maintenance and twelve hugs a day for growth, so why not be hugged all night? As you snuggle under the weighted blanket, the gentle pressure on your body triggers the release of serotonin, a neurotransmitter that calms the mind and body, making it easier to fall asleep and stay asleep. The added weight also has a profound impact on the body's production of melatonin, the hormone responsible for regulating our sleep-wake cycles. As a result, weighted blankets have been shown to improve sleep quality and reduce restlessness and anxiety. They come in different weights, as there's not necessarily one weight that suits all. Even in the summer I will have it on me over a thin top sheet, as it's not too hot. It's like a cuddle from a big bear and it immediately relaxes me into a solid sleep.

Blackout blinds

Blackout blinds are fab, and you can even get travel ones now that you stick to the wall with Velcro. Or you can wear an eye mask if you're stimulated by light. We leave the hall light on for my five-year-old in case she stirs or needs to go to the loo in the night, and even that sliver of light under the door gets me looking around the room, so I sleep with an eye mask on.

Earplugs

As a mummy, I'm hypersensitive to my child's energy and wearing my earplugs has never prevented me from waking if she's woken up crying, been sick or had a nightmare, but it does stop my partner's snoring and heavy breathing driving me mad. I have reusable ones that are made from silicone. These are the best that I've tried, and I have tried many earplugs over the years. They also feel the most hygienic because I can wash them. It also means, in the summer months, I can have the window open and not hear the milkman clunking along at 5am.

On Awakening

What you do when you wake up in the morning also affects how you sleep that night!

This first hour after waking should be a digital-free hour. No emails, no social media, no checking the news or catching up on work. Think of your body as like a car; you would never turn the engine on and go straight into fifth gear. What would happen if you did? You would burn out your clutch and the engine would eventually break down . . . That's what turning on your phone first thing in the morning does to the body. We're immediately on high alert and in fight or flight mode. We need to warm up the engine and ease through the lower gears before we hit fifth gear – i.e. the demands of life.

Journalling

I mentioned journalling back in Week 2, but making it a part of your wake-up routine is where it comes into its own. Keep a pad and pen next to your bed, and each morning as soon as you open your eyes, free-write for two to three pages. We often wake up with a negative mindset or with a 'woulda, coulda, shoulda' narrative running on a loop. Free-writing gives you the opportunity to dump all this on the page. Like any poison, it is better out than in. It also allows you to release certain things lurking in the conscious or subconscious mind. As you grow with this practice, you may be surprised at what comes up, and that is its beauty. It's a non-judgemental space, it's pretty much free, and you can take it anywhere with you. I am in my twentieth year of this practice, and it's been my saving grace during life's most challenging times.

Gratitude list

> 'Gratitude unlocks the fullness of life . . . It turns denial into acceptance, chaos into order, confusion into clarity . . . It turns problems into gifts, failures into success, and mistakes into important events. Gratitude makes sense of our past, brings peace for today and creates a vision for tomorrow.'
>
> Melody Beattie

After journalling, do your gratitude list. Write three things you are grateful for in the present and three things you are grateful for in the future, but write them both in the present tense. This act of not merely thinking thanks but writing them down is powerful. There is a great deal of scientific evidence to support how a gratitude list can vastly benefit your health.

A 2015 study found some impressive insights. Not only did a gratitude list improve sleep quality and enhance mood, but the patients who were making the gratitude list had lower inflammation markers and had a more significant heart variability than the patients who were not keeping a gratitude list.[36]

Detox and revive

Next, simply get up and get moving! Move in a way that gets your heart rate up and gets you a little sweaty, whether it be jogging, dancing, HIIT, Zumba, yoga, Tabata, or whatever you like to do most. We all know that dopamine is a feel-good hormone, but did you know that exercise releases serotonin, dopamine and epinephrine? Stephanie Fine Sasse, a trained Harvard University and Oregon Health and Sciences University researcher, explains that dopamine 'plays a role in learning and memory formation and reward, particularly making you feel good. We all desire to step into our day with that feel-good factor rather than feeling the need to reach for another coffee. An excellent tip to enable that daily commitment is to lay your workout clothes out the night before, so you step into them as you get out of bed.'

Nourish from nature

Getting morning sunlight (but never look directly at the sun) is excellent for getting a dose of vitamin D and a brilliant tool for setting your body clock. This needs to be done outside, so whether you go for a 10- to 20-minute walk in nature or around your block, stand in your garden or on your balcony, you need to get the eye connecting with the direct light. You can't do this through a window, as the stimulus is fifty times less effective.

According to Dr Andrew Huberman, tenured Professor of Neurobiology and Ophthalmology at Stanford University School of Medicine, much of how we perform in the day and how we sleep at night is determined by how much daylight we get in that first hour.

Huberman says on his podcast *Hubermanlab*, 'When we wake up, our eyes open. If we're in a dark room, there isn't enough light to trigger the correct timing of this cortisol and melatonin rhythm. At daybreak, when the sun is low in the sky, there's a particular contrast between yellows and blues, and that triggers the activation of cortisol. Once the sun is overhead, the quality of light shifts so that you miss this opportunity to time the cortisol pulse.'

Don't stress, I'm not asking you to join the 5am club. Simply go outside as early as you can after sunrise for as long as you can.

Movement is key in the morning, as far as I am concerned, as it literally gets the whole body moving, even the colon. You want to poop *before* your morning coffee, not rely on it to empty your bowels. Movement will aid this. Also, when you poop well, you sleep well.

I know being outside isn't possible for everybody, but when you can, embrace it. Even in the cooler months, my partner, our daughter and I will sit on the balcony, or we'll sit in the lounge with the balcony doors open with rugs on us and have a breakfast picnic. It's nice to feel the fresh air, even if it's quite chilly (when you live in the North of England, it's more often than not chilly). And it will help you sleep well that evening.

If none of this has convinced you of the importance of sleep, let's take it back to the pioneers of modern health, the Ancient Greeks, who are renowned for their natural and holistic approach to medicine and their emphasis on rational thinking. They knew how much sleep was imperative to life's existence, so much so that they even had a God for it: Hypnos.

In his treatise *Breaths*, Hippocrates highlighted sleep as a critical factor for maintaining health. He described how sleep reduces body temperature and slows blood flow to the brain, supporting the body's restorative functions. Hippocrates is known as the 'Father of Medicine', as the Ancient Greek physician's teachings laid the foundation for modern medical ethics and practice. His influence persists today, as newly qualified doctors in the UK and around the world often pledge a version of the Hippocratic Oath, committing to uphold ethical standards in patient care. So, I invite you to rethink sleep, to honour it for all the work it's doing for your body and mind. Think of yourself as a Formula 1 car, a very expensive, finely tuned vehicle, and then think of your bed as your pit stop where all the maintenance takes place for the next lap around the track, the next day of your life.

Sometimes the most beneficial things are the basics.

> 'I'm a doer and a busy woman. I realised I was popping every pill going, but was not prioritising sleep. I was the woman who took her laptop to bed to check in on other time zones within my company. When I stopped doing this and started a sleep prep practice (it was hard at first), my period levelled out and my sex life got better, as there were no longer three of us in a bed: me, my husband and my laptop.'
>
> Mary

Week 7. Lowering the Toxic Burden

In Week 5, I stated that hydration is key to fertility, and it is one of the foundational pillars of health. I will shout from the rooftops for as long as people will listen about how important it is to clean up the basics: sleep, hydration, food, movement, and how we respond to stress, before we pop the pills. These foundations must be established before we add the next layers, before we start to try to conceive naturally or before we embark on IVF. I say this because so much can be done for free or at a fairly low cost.

We drink water every day, so we need to look at the quality of the water we're drinking. OK, I'm just going to say it and let the naysayers come after me: I'm not a fan of tap water. And can you believe it, neither are my cats.

Many clients say they can't afford a water filter or to splash out (pardon the pun) on a whole-house water filter system.

But may I suggest, you can. There are under-the-sink filters that cost less than £100 and that you can fit yourself in less than 10 minutes. Plus, the added bonus is this water is not stored in plastic, and it's not just for drinking but readily available to cook with too.

It's Week 7 now and you have hopefully gone at least four weeks without any alcohol. You will have also eaten less processed food, and therefore will have a little more money spare. We have removed these expenditures and can replace them with one that will support your journey. Think about it: ladies, all you need to do is give up your toxic acrylic or shellac nail treatment for a month or two and you can get an under-the-sink filter system; give it up for a year and you can purchase a whole-house water filter system.

By choosing where to invest your money like this, you will be lowering your exposure to a whole army of toxins that can disrupt your hormones, which can affect not only your fertility but also your overall health – and the health of your child-in-waiting when they arrive.

Water

I am fully aware that I am blessed to even have running water in my home and I'm also aware that, living in the UK, I am no longer at risk of life-threatening infections, such as typhoid and cholera. I am very thankful for this, as I have spent time volunteering in a refugee camp where this is not the case. But – and this is a big but in my mind – what I'm also aware of is the decline of fertility in the Western world and that often, when I turn on my tap at home, the water that comes pouring out smells of chlorine and can have a metallic taste. Therefore, I use a countertop filtration system. If you have ever drunk water straight from a fresh stream, you will have noted that it's an experience far from what you get from your glass of tap water at home.

I am a firm believer that we have been chemicallised to such a degree that we are now exposed to different kinds of health risk than we were a hundred years ago. We are living longer but getting sicker younger. What's changed? A lot!

Our drinking water is a great example of how our modern world is so far removed from nature. It's not just the chlorine, the limescale or the fluoride in our tap water. If you live in an old property and you have lead pipes, your water has to flow through those pipes. The water companies have to treat soft and hard water areas with different chemicals. For example, if you live in a soft water area, you're more likely to have lead in your water, as limescale in hard water can coat the inside of pipes and prevent lead from dissolving into the water. In soft water areas, the chemical orthophosphate is added to the water to prevent lead leaching into it.

One common misconception is that drinking water is 'safe' if the amount of lead is less than the amount stipulated in the drinking water standards. Please note, however, that the World Health Organization has stated that there is no safe limit for lead, and also note that water companies are often fined for not keeping to the safe levels recommended.

A number of studies have been done to see how phosphates affect the human body and the jury is still out. Much of it balances on the word 'safe' and, just as certain chemicals such as lead have been deemed 'safe' in the past and are now deemed 'not safe', hence why many people choose to use a water filter to remove it.

Research suggests that high concentrations of orthophosphate in drinking water may disrupt the balance of gut microbiota, leading to digestive issues and inflammation. Inflammation, we know, has a direct link to fertility in both males and females. Furthermore, the presence of orthophosphate has been linked to oxidative stress and cellular damage, potentially accelerating the ageing of tissues and organs (here, think of egg quality and how doctors always talk about 'old eggs').

Reverse osmosis is one of the most common and effective methods for removing phosphates in drinking water. It can remove between 93 and 99% of phosphates, depending on the type of treatment unit.

Even if you have great water pipes and a great water supplier that hasn't been fined of late, what about microplastics?

Microplastics have been found in up to 72% of tap water samples in European nations, including the UK. Many researchers and the media have highlighted the damaging effects these microplastics are having on our fertility, weight and hormones.

Next up, synthetic hormones. Men and women who are vehemently trying to improve their fertility don't want to be drinking tap water contaminated with the contraceptive pill. Research indicates that exposure to synthetic hormones from contraceptive pills in water sources may interfere with the hormonal balance in men especially, leading to decreased sperm quality and quantity. These disruptions can impact various aspects of male reproductive health, including sperm motility and morphology, both of which are, incidentally, the most common low results in sperm analysis.

This is just one aspect that has had the spotlight shone on it; however, think of all the other drugs that people take: paracetamol, anti-inflammatories, antidepressants, and then recreational drugs, such as cocaine. These have all been found in tap water.

Every year the Drinking Water Inspectorate brings to court water companies in the UK for failure to supply water fit for human consumption.

This is just one example in recent years:

'Summary of the High Park Chlorate event involving the incorrect storage of sodium hypochlorite resulting in chlorate above the WHO recommended guidelines in drinking water.

'During May 2018, 48 consumers in Sussex were potentially exposed to a level of sodium chlorate in their drinking water above the maximum World Health Organisation recommended concentration of 700μg/l. The maximum concentration detected was 994μg/l.

'[Southern Water] failed to store the chemical in the correct manner... As such, the sodium hypochlorite which is used to maintain a residual chlorination degraded and formed sodium chlorate. A toxicological assessment determined that in this instance the actions by the Company to reduce the time consumers were exposed meant that the likelihood of any harm was remote.

'Sodium chlorate is not visible in the concentrations involved and does not have a taste or smell. Therefore, consumers would have been unaware of any issues and would have continued to consume their drinking water as normal.'

The 'investigation found that the risk assessment carried out by Southern Water on site repeatedly failed to adequately control the likelihood of degradation of sodium hypochlorite, resulting in this event.'

What is chlorate?

Chlorate is a chemical compound found in certain water sources and food products that has been linked to potential disruptions in thyroid function and hormone levels. Tap water, however, is the main source of chlorate in our diet, possibly contributing up to 60% of chronic chlorate exposure in infants. Studies suggest that exposure to chlorate may interfere with the thyroid and its ability to produce essential hormones, and as you will know by now, it's vital that the thyroid is functioning optimally for fertility.

I believe that it is crucial to be aware of potential sources of chlorate exposure and to take steps to minimise its effects on thyroid function and hormone levels to support optimal reproductive health. Start to think about what is really coming out of your tap; it may look clear, but that certainly doesn't mean it's pure.

Please don't drop this book and run to the supermarket to get your favourite plastic bottle of water, however. Because . . . Yes, you've guessed it, I'm not a fan of plastic bottles of water.

It's not just the plastic and what it's doing to our planet. We are all told not to drink bottled water if it has been left in the car or the sun for too long at the beach. Why? Because sunlight causes BPA (bisphenol A) and PET (polyethylene terephthalate) to leak into the water.

If the European Union has banned some types of phthalates in children's toys and the use of BPA in plastic baby bottles, why are they not banned for adults?

A 2017 UK study found that BPA was detected in the urine of 86% of participants.[37]

A recent 2023 research initiative 'measured chemicals in people's bodies in Europe and detected BPA in the urine of 92% of adult participants from eleven European countries.'[38]

Even if your bottle of water does say it is BPA-free, it's still plastic and will still contain chemicals that make plastic. All the company is saying is that this plastic bottle does not contain BPA; it is not telling you what chemical it has replaced it with that is not yet banned, and don't forget that they have chosen this other chemical purely because it is similar to BPA and will therefore most likely affect the body in the same way. This is when PET is more commonly used, so what have the people in white coats been saying about this chemical?

Back in 2009, concerns were already being raised and *Environmental Health Perspectives* published a paper that stated, 'The evidence suggests that PET bottles may yield endocrine disruptors under conditions of common use, particularly with prolonged storage and elevated temperature.'[39]

BPA and PET are just two chemicals you may or may not be familiar with. However, there are many more. Did you know that there are more than 16,000 chemicals used in plastics manufacturing, and over 1,000 industrial chemicals used today are thought to be endocrine disruptors?

Think also about the long road your bottle of water has taken from source to consumer. It needs to be pulled from the source, then taken to a factory to be bottled up and then the bottle has to be sealed and then stored in a warehouse. Next step the bottle has to be transported to your local supermarket warehouse and then redistributed again to the store. Finally, it is placed on the supermarket shelf under many lights. You may argue that safety procedures are implemented, but we all know that things don't always go according to plan. What's to say that your plastic bottle of water that is doubled-wrapped in more plastic was not left in the sun while some storage issues were sorted out at your local shop? I have gone into many shops where the plastic bottles that are stored on the shelf and not in the fridge are warm to touch. But even if it's cold, was it warm before it was put in the fridge? To my mind, it's not worth the risk.

Why do I have an issue with drinking these chemicals? Let the specialists explain if I have not convinced you so far.

According to the Endocrine Society, 'Plastics contain and leach hazardous chemicals, including endocrine-disrupting chemicals (EDCs) that threaten human health . . . EDCs are chemicals that disturb the body's hormone systems and can cause cancer, diabetes, reproductive disorders, and neurological impairments of developing foetuses and children. The report describes a wealth of evidence supporting direct cause-and-effect links between the toxic chemical additives in plastics and specific health impacts to the endocrine system.'

So, if you must drink bottled water, please purchase it in a glass bottle for the sake of the environment and your fertility.

While tap water in the UK and USA generally meets 'safety' standards (I always put that word in quotation marks, because what was deemed safe twenty years ago, ten years ago or even a few years ago may not be deemed safe today or in the future), there have been numerous studies that have raised concerns regarding microplastic exposure and its potential impact on fertility.

In women, exposure to EDCs in tap water may contribute to

unexplained infertility by affecting ovulation, menstrual regularity and hormone levels.

PFAS are another chemical found in our water. PFAS exposure may cause menopause to occur two years earlier in women, according to a new study published in the Endocrine Society's *Journal of Clinical Endocrinology & Metabolism*.

For men, EDCs in tap water can impact sperm quality and quantity, potentially leading to reduced fertility. It is crucial to consider the potential effects of tap water quality on reproductive health and explore ways to minimise exposure to EDCs to support overall fertility and hormonal balance.[40]

According to a study by Mount Sinai researchers, exposure to chemicals commonly found in drinking water and everyday household products may result in reduced fertility in women by as much as 40%.[41]

Studies have shown that exposure to BPA can have significant negative effects on fertility in both men and women. Here's a closer look at the research:

Effect on male fertility:

- Several studies have found that higher levels of BPA in the body are associated with reduced sperm quality, including lower sperm count, motility and morphology.

- One study of over 300 men found that those with the highest BPA levels had a 23% lower sperm concentration and 10% lower sperm vitality compared to men with the lowest BPA exposure.
- BPA is believed to disrupt the endocrine system and interfere with the production and function of reproductive hormones like testosterone, which are crucial for normal sperm development.

Effect on female fertility:

- BPA exposure has been linked to an increased risk of miscarriage and other adverse reproductive outcomes in women.
- One study found that women with the highest BPA levels had over 2 times the risk of miscarriage compared to those with the lowest exposures.
- BPA may interfere with normal ovarian function, egg maturation, and implantation of the embryo, all of which are essential for successful pregnancy.
- Some research suggests BPA may also increase the risk of polycystic ovary syndrome (PCOS), a leading cause of infertility in women.

Most humans can only go three days without water before they die, so we can see just how important it is. Water is the first thing that I encourage people to invest in, so find a solution that is financially comfortable for you.

Also, when out and about, always avoid ice, as we don't know what type of water it's made from.

Tinned Cans

BPA and PFAS aren't just found in our water.

Is your tin of beans for your weekend English breakfast or tin of tomatoes for your favourite pasta dish contributing to your toxic build-up?

BPA is commonly used in the lining of metal food and beverage cans to prevent corrosion and extend shelf life. However, numerous studies have shown that BPA can leach into the food and beverages contained in these cans, posing a significant health risk. BPA was once used in till receipts but, due to health concerns, many supermarkets stopped using it as far back as 2010. Supermarket chains such as Lidl replaced their BPA receipts years ago, as the shiny BPA coating cannot be recycled and there was also a rise in concern for the cashiers' health.

Many companies, such as Coca-Cola, Campbell's and Heinz, have taken steps to remove BPA from the lining of their cans in response to growing public concern. Additionally, several countries, including Canada, the European Union and China, have banned the use of BPA in certain consumer products, particularly those intended for infants and young children. This is due to the mounting evidence that BPA exposure, even at low levels, can interfere with normal hormonal function and development, potentially leading to reproductive problems, including reduced sperm quality, altered menstrual cycles and increased risk of miscarriage.

The effects of BPA on fertility appear to be dose-dependent, with higher exposures generally causing greater impairment. Given the ubiquity of BPA in our food, personal care and household products, reducing exposure is an important step for couples looking to conceive. Minimising the use of tinned foods, plastic containers and other BPA-containing items can help lower overall body burden of this concerning chemical.

Even when companies have removed BPA from their tins, what have they replaced it with? There still has to be some kind of inner coating to form a barrier between the food and the aluminium can. For example, the acidity of tinned tomatoes would cause aluminium to leach into your food.

A great option here is to buy dried foods, such as beans, and then store them in glass jars. Also, simply use less tinned food; the more food you cook from scratch, the lower your exposure to 'forever chemicals' will be.

We want to 'Stay away from BPA [and PFAS]'.

Bathing

Yes, bath and shower water counts too.

If 70% of what we put on our skin is absorbed into our body and our skin is our biggest organ, it makes sense not to bathe or shower in chemicallised water. Many people scoff when I suggest this.

HRT is the buzzword of the moment in female wellbeing. It has revolutionised the menopause for many women and given them a whole new lease of life, as it can regulate hormones and support symptoms. One of the ways to take the prescribed hormones is to use a gel or spray on the skin. Therefore, if this gel or spray changes a woman's hormones so significantly that her menopausal symptoms diminish, this is indisputable proof that what we apply topically to our skin can and does have a direct effect on our health.

Therefore, I suggest you explore either a whole-house filter system or a simple attachment to the shower or bath, which you can get from as little as £20. This is a small step that can make a big difference to your toxic burden.

SPF

Is SPF protecting you or is it yet another obstacle in the way of you becoming a parent?

While I encourage people to wear sunscreen, even those who are working indoors if they have windows, I do not encourage anyone to slather harmful chemicals onto their skin. Many sunscreens contain chemicals that are toxic to the ecosystem that is the human body and also toxic to aquatic life (if you are on holiday or blessed to live near water).

Some of the chemicals that I discuss here are actually banned in a number of countries. Yes, banned! Why? Because they are harmful to sea life and coral (i.e. some of these chemicals bleach the coral) and human health. Hawaii and Palau have banned the use of these harmful chemicals in SPF products due to their detrimental impact on marine ecosystems and human health. Even a number of water parks have banned them in Mexico.

A study published in 2019 found that, after a single application, seven chemicals commonly found in sunscreens can be absorbed into the bloodstream at levels that exceed safety thresholds.[42]

'What is most alarming about these findings is that chemicals are absorbing into the body in significant amounts and the ingredients have not been fully tested for safety,' said David Andrews, a senior scientist for the Environmental Working Group (EWG), a consumer organisation that advocates for sunscreen safety.

The toxic chemicals in SPF products disrupt human hormones because they are endocrine disruptors. Chemicals like oxybenzone and octinoxate, commonly found in sunscreens, have been linked to hormonal imbalances and adverse health effects. Oxybenzone has even been found in breast milk.

One study found that 'Twenty-seven out of the 79 human breast milk samples analysed (34%) contained UV-Fs. High concentrations were determined for oxybenzone and its metabolites.'[43]

These are the main chemicals in sunscreen that you want to avoid, and which you definitely want to avoid using on your child:

1. Oxybenzone (Benzophenone-3): Known to disrupt hormone levels, particularly oestrogen (it mimics it, and potentially affects thyroid function and we need your

thyroid in top working order for fertility optimisation). It can also interfere with testosterone production and disrupt adrenal hormones. This is one chemical to definitely step away from.
2. Octinoxate (Ethylhexyl Methoxycinnamate): Associated with interference in thyroid hormone production and endocrine function, leading to hormonal imbalances once again.
3. Homosalate: Research suggests homosalate may mimic oestrogen in the body, potentially disrupting the endocrine system and affecting hormone regulation.
4. Octocrylene: Linked to hormone disruption, especially impacting oestrogen and thyroid hormones. If it can bleach coral reefs, it must be strong.

You can see which sunscreens may be of concern by screening them on the EWG website or by using apps such as Think Dirty or Yuka.

Safe alternatives to consider are mineral-based sunscreens containing zinc oxide or titanium dioxide, which provide effective UV protection without the harmful side effects of chemical filters. These mineral sunscreens are considered reef-safe, biodegradable and less likely to cause hormone disruption or skin irritation.

Yet another downside to chemical sunscreens is that you are advised to wait 20 to 30 minutes before exposing the skin to the sun for full protection, but with a mineral sunscreen you get instant protection, so it's a double win.

You don't have to spend a fortune on mineral-based sunscreens either, but many out there are significantly overpriced because the beauty industry knows that 'clean' beauty is big bucks, so I encourage you to look for sunscreens from independent brands, which you can get for around £10.

Please do your research, as even I have been caught out in the past. Many brands claim that they are mineral 'based' and legally, yes, they may be mineral 'based', but the BASE is not the whole picture and it does not mean it is toxic-chemical free. It may still contain homosalate and octocrylene, as these two chemicals have had the least bad press coverage, so are not in the forefront of consumers' minds. So always, always look at the full list of ingredients.

There are some good companies out there that have complete transparency and even display their comprehensive test analysis online for you to view. The EWG has lots on their website and you can also use your Think Dirty or Yukka app to find a clean and sun-safe SPF.

Tampons

One would think that tampons and sanitary towels would legally not be allowed to contain any toxins; especially tampons, seeing that they are inserted internally. I remember way back in my first year of university (about thirty years ago – yes, as many years as some of you have been on this planet), a boyfriend who was far wiser than myself and his peers at the time told me not to use tampons or even disposable sanitary towels and to use a piece of cut-up bathroom towel instead. I tried to do so when he was around and then used the disposable ones when he wasn't around. I have since told him I was wrong and he was right, but it was a world where talc on babies' bums and vaginas was still encouraged in hospitals and we were all loving spray deodorants.

We have moved on since then, yet three decades later many conventional tampons still contain concerning chemicals, like chlorine, dioxins and synthetic fragrances (all will be revealed in the next section on chemical fragrance) that can disrupt the delicate endocrine system.

When these tampons are used internally, the chemicals can be readily absorbed through the thin, permeable lining of the vagina and enter the bloodstream. Think about how much thinner your skin is inside than outside. In fact, the skin inside the vagina is approximately 3–5 times thinner than the skin on the external genitalia and other areas of the body.

This extreme thinness of the vaginal tissue means it is more vulnerable to absorbing chemicals. The vaginal lining also has a rich blood supply directly underneath, which provides a direct route for chemicals to enter the bloodstream and circulate throughout the body. Also, think of what is close to your vagina – the cervix and your ovaries. Why place anything toxic close to this environment? This delicate vulnerability is a key reason why the use of tampons containing chemicals like dioxins and fragrances can be such a fertility disruptor.

Just as my old boyfriend, the wise owl from uni, pleaded with me, I plead with you to choose an alternative for your bleed time. Luckily for you, you don't need to cut up your bath towels, as there are now several safer alternatives on the market. Organic cotton tampons, menstrual cups, reusable cloth pads and some, but not all, period pants. Be careful and do your research when purchasing period pants, as many contain chemicals like PFAS, and you know these are 'forever chemicals', which can disrupt hormones. Other potential toxins include phthalates, which affect reproductive health. Most high street chemists and supermarkets sell organic feminine hygiene products and they aren't that much more expensive either. Always look out for the Soil Association label, as this certification is hard to earn and you know you will be purchasing a trusted brand.

Skincare and perfume (fragrance)

What's in your beauty bag may not be so beautiful at all.

I love to smell beautiful. Smell is one of the five senses that I am very sensitive to and affected by. Let's just say I have a strong sense of smell.

A fragrance can have such a positive effect on my mood. It can lift me up, and it can make me feel stronger, more assertive, more relaxed. I have a fragrance for work, one for social and one for when I do my public speaking, where I feel I need that extra level of support. However, my fragrance may be a little different from yours. A fragrance full of chemicals will have a whole different effect on me. It can make me cough, make my eyes sting and leave me feeling heavy-headed. I don't even need to be wearing it. We have all walked past that person on the street who seems to have bathed in perfume or aftershave, and we start to cough. These effects got me thinking, and I started investigating fragrances at the start of my own fertility journey. What I found out was even more shocking than the SPF revelations.

Above I showed just how much effect what we put on our skin can have on our body through the example of topical HRT. It's the same for shower gels, perfumes, makeup and many other beauty products.

These products are frequently fragranced. The issue with a lot of fragrances is that the perfume makers are not legally obliged to state the 'magic' formula, so often we don't know exactly what we are spraying around our rooms or on our bodies. Many are filled with a number of 'forever chemicals', which can damage the vulnerable ovarian follicles and the development of your precious eggs. Often women who are struggling with fertility have a low follicle count, so protecting this is imperative to your fertility journey. So, it's good to know how many toxins you may be piling onto your skin and into your body and, more importantly, what to do about it.

People often say to me, 'A little of something won't hurt you', and I agree. But it's not a little, is it? Because a little of something plus a little of something else and a little of something else again builds up to a lot. Hence why we are now seeing evidence of phthalates and 'forever chemicals' in urine, breast milk and even in newborn babies.

The EWG found that the average woman used twelve products a day, which added up to 168 chemicals; that's 61,320 chemicals a year. So if you have been wearing makeup since you were sixteen and you are now thirty-five, that's over a million chemicals that your body was not born to deal with. Let's note that the twelve products a day was also an average, and if some women don't wear makeup at all, that raises the average significantly for those who do.

These phthalates also disrupt the ovaries' ability to produce oestrogen and progesterone. Therefore, if we have a high toxic load from mascara, face cream, toner, face masks, lipsticks, hairspray, dry shampoo, body lotion and deodorant – there's more, but you get my drift – this burden is going to contribute to hormone imbalance. The body's skin is your biggest organ, but because it's on the outside we often forget this.

Legally, beauty companies are not required to stipulate exactly what ingredients they have used, and they can just state 'fragrance' or 'perfume' on a label. But what does this actually mean?

As a postnatal doula, I always encourage my new parents not to wear any kind of fragrance so the baby can get used to their natural scent, but also so they are not transferring any chemicals onto the delicate thin skin of their precious newborn.

I will now break down why I want you to swap your favourite scent for a natural alternative.

Words to look out for and stay away from:

Musk ketone

The chemical fragrance compound musk, which is used to create a 'clean' or 'fresh' scent and is present in many gender-neutral fragrances, has been found to be toxic to the brain, liver and lungs, as well as aquatic life. Exposure to musk has also been linked to gynaecological issues like ovarian failure and infertility. It's in nearly all male fragrances. More research needs to be done on human studies, but as I have highlighted, we really do need to investigate the effect of lifestyle on sperm, due to the dramatic decline in sperm results in recent decades.

Animal studies have found that exposure to musk ketone can lead to reduced sperm count, decreased sperm motility, and morphological abnormalities in sperm, which are all common in human male infertility. Musk ketone has also been shown to have anti-androgenic effects, meaning it can block or reduce the activity of male sex hormones like testosterone. Having an imbalance in testosterone levels and function can impair overall semen production.

It's not a pretty picture for women either. One study concludes that 'nitro musks could be disruptors of the hypothalamic-ovarian hormone pathway'.[44]

A peer-review study of relevant literature up to August 2020 was published to determine whether perfumes and colognes can affect people's health, and its findings will be of interest to you chaps especially.

'Phthalates affect male reproductive development by inhibiting androgen biosynthesis.

'There is a relationship between urinary monoethyl phthalate (MEP) concentration and sperm DNA damage and between urinary monobutyl phthalate (MBP) and monobenzyl phthalate (MBzP) concentrations with decreased sperm motility. [Normal speak: this means that the more 'forever chemicals' found in you, the less likely your sperm is going to swim in the right direction.]

'Exposure to parabens can seriously damage sperm DNA, male reproductive health and the reproductive system of male animals.'[45] [Note that DNA fragmentation of sperm is often cited as a main factor in implantation failure and recurrent miscarriage.]

General guidance is to limit exposure to musk fragrances for men trying to conceive.

Benzyl acetate

This chemical has been banned or restricted in many countries due to its toxicity, but there are currently no such restrictions in the United States. The fact that it may be 'less toxic than many other chemicals' does not negate the potential risks, as the interactions and byproducts formed when these chemicals are combined can create even more harmful compounds, such as methylene chloride.

Methylene chloride, aka paint stripper. Methylene chloride has now been banned in the UK for personal sale and use. So I beg the question, why is it still used in any industry that sells a product for cosmetic use?

Its known side effects are dizziness, drowsiness, irritation, and adverse skin disorders that may even contribute to types of cancer. However, it's still allowed to be used for perfumes.

I personally use a vegan brand of perfume. I'm not a vegan but it is a brand that omits toxic chemicals and replaces them with essential oils. I have been using these perfumes for six years now and they have the added benefit of also having a longer-lasting smell. Often, I will pop on a cardigan or a jacket that I wore a week or so ago and it still smells wonderful. This simple remove and replace means you do not have to compromise, plus it happens to be cheaper than some popular brands and also less costly to the body. It's a triple win.

Where cosmetics and skincare are concerned, check your apps again and see what you are willing to swap in and out. A simple swap is a natural soap bar instead of body wash. Go back to the old soap on a rope or a soap bag so it doesn't end up being a mushy mess in the shower. Natural soap bags double up as an exfoliant, can be washed and reused, and can be bought for as little as £3, so they are a great investment.

Makeup and creams: where you can, look for ones in glass jars to avoid plastic leaching into the product. Some companies even do refills.

You don't need to replace everything at once. By slowly removing and replacing your products as you run out, you will lower your daily chemical exposure. It all counts.

> 'It was a huge turning point for me working on this week, when I realised no matter what I was putting into my body – wonderful healthy foods, good fats, vitamins – if I didn't work on my home environment and what I was putting onto my skin and therefore into my body, things would be affected! I'd been lighting candles, spraying room sprays and perfume all over me and into my environment!! I was using skincare that contained hormone distributors without even knowing it! Liberty taught me about the toxic load, talking me through everything in detail and helped me remove these, recommending wonderful affordable natural products that would support my journey and make me feel good without interfering with my fertility. I switched to a mineral-based daily

sunscreen and changed all my beauty products – and it made such a difference. I started to not only feel better and look better, but it completely supported my journey as I was pregnant within months in my forties. Everyone's journey and experience is different, but I know this discovery and practice made a huge difference to me and helped me to achieve my goal.'

Hollie

Week 8. Cleaning Up Your Home Environment

This is a great week to remove and replace.

The aim of the previous chapter and this chapter is to raise your awareness of the effects of toxins on your health and fertility and encourage you to slowly remove and replace certain everyday things in your life that are not serving you well. We have to live our lives, and fertility is stressful enough as it is, but these simple swaps can help lower the stress on your hormones and your body in general.

Plastic Utensils

When it comes to plastic utensils, it's basic common sense. If you heat something up to such a high temperature and then place plastic into it, it's going to melt. I wish I could show you some of the plastic spatulas clients have sent me photographs of over the years, because they are tragic. One person had had the same spatula all his married life of nineteen years!

No one wants melted plastic juice in their stir fry or as the base of their shepherd's pie.

Opt instead for stainless steel and wooden cooking tools. They're non-toxic and they're also more durable, so they won't melt or warp like plastic can and often does under intense heat over the years.

Cookware

Avoid, where you can, non-stick – especially old-school Teflon – types of cookware. And especially non-stick frying pans. Look up the brand that's in your kitchen cupboard and see what it's made from. Most common types of cookware contain harmful chemicals and coatings that can leach into your food, many of which have been found to pose serious health risks and are, yes, you've guessed it, big endocrine disruptors. If you've had your non-stick pan for years, it may have a toxic chemical coating that has since been banned.

Non-stick pans are often coated in 'forever chemicals'. When these pans are heated, the chemical coating can release toxic fumes into the air and the chemicals can leach into your food.

Instead, opt for cookware made of safer natural materials like stainless steel, cast iron or ceramic. These alternatives don't have the same toxic chemical concerns, plus they can withstand high heat without degrading. For a truly non-stick surface, look for pans coated with a mineral-based ceramic glaze. Cast-iron, stainless steel and ceramic non-stick pans may be more expensive than some coated pans, but they're likely to last longer, as well as being safer. We actually have a set from our grandparents. Look on eBay for second-hand pots and pans, and many discount stores often sell luxury brands such as Le Creuset at a discounted price.

Tea Bags

Not all tea bags are nasty, but some contain plastic, so please do read the labels of your favourite brands. You could even email the company and ask if it is not clear. Or if you are reading or listening to this in the UK or the USA, there are plenty of websites that have already done the work for you and have an up-to-date list of the most commonly consumed teas and if they contain plastic. Be thorough, as even within a single brand's range the use of plastic can vary.

Why do I loathe plastic in your tea? According to a 2019 study, stewing a plastic tea bag at a brewing temperature of 95°C releases around 11.6 billion microplastics and 3.1 billion nanoplastics into a single cup.[46] This cup of tea no longer sounds so cosy and innocent but more than a little gross.

Polypropylene (PP) and nylon (the latter often found in premium and high-end brands of tea) are the most common plastics used in tea bags. Both have been found to have an effect on hormonal disruption and may contribute to reduced sperm quality, count and motility. Some research indicates these compounds, like all the other endocrine disruptors, can mimic oestrogen, therefore creating a hormone imbalance.

So, my advice is switch to loose teas or tea bags that are natural and unbleached, and, if not, simply limit your tea intake and increase your filtered water intake. Or make your own tea. Chai tea is a great one for lowering inflammation and balancing hormones, and, in addition, it is a warming tea for the ladies, which is good for fertility. You could make fresh mint teas, traditional nettle tea, even dip you toe into Ayurveda and soak fennel seeds for fennel tea. And let's not forget good old lemon and ginger tea. There are so many options, so you don't have to miss out just because you are skipping the toxic tea bag.

Washing Fruits and Veg (vegetables)

I did a reel on Instagram on this topic and it went viral. Unfortunately, not really for the content, but because I said veg rather than vegetables and because of my Northern accent, some people thought I said vag! I *never* say vag, always vagina. Anyhow, why did I do a post on washing and/or soaking your fruit and vegetables? Firstly, it removes dirt and bugs, and this is helpful if you buy fresh produce that still has soil and a few creepy crawlies on it (insects are a sign of good-quality produce, as long as it's not riddled with them). And, secondly, it can remove pesticides. Some fruit, for example supermarket strawberries, can contain high levels of pesticides due to their porous nature. This is why a lot of books will tell you to go fully organic when it comes to fresh produce. But I understand that's not financially viable for everyone, especially if you have a large family, and it's also hard to find everything organic if you are shopping locally. For example, where I live I can only source organic carrots, organic broccoli, organic cucumber and sometimes organic apples. Everything else I would have to order online, which would be at greater expense.

So, what do I do and what do I encourage?

Know your produce.

Let me introduce to you the Dirty Dozen and the Clean Fifteen.

Being in the know is at the core of why I wrote this book. If you don't know, you simply don't know, and then you are unable to make an informed choice. Knowing what is considered the safest non-organic produce, and what to buy organic if you can, takes a lot of stress out of your shopping and food choices.

The Dirty Dozen and the Clean Fifteen are lists compiled annually and placed online, with downloadable versions also available, which are handy for when you are shopping. In the UK this list is compiled by Pesticide Action Network (PAN), and in the USA it is by the Environmental Working Group (EWG). These lists aim to provide shoppers like you and me with a guide to which fruits and vegetables tend to have the highest and lowest levels of pesticide residues.

The Dirty Dozen. The name says it all; this list consists of the twelve fruits and vegetables found to have the highest concentrations of pesticide residues.

At the time of writing this book in 2024, the current PAN UK Dirty Dozen is as follows:

1. Spinach
2. Strawberries
3. Kale
4. Nectarines
5. Apples
6. Grapes
7. Bell peppers
8. Cherries

9. Peaches
10. Pears
11. Celery
12. Tomatoes

The 2024 EWG Dirty Dozen

1. Strawberries
2. Spinach
3. Kale
4. Nectarines
5. Apples
6. Grapes
7. Bell peppers
8. Cherries
9. Peaches
10. Pears
11. Celery
12. Tomatoes

The 2024 EWG (USA) Clean Fifteen

1. Avocados
2. Sweetcorn
3. Pineapples
4. Onions
5. Papaya
6. Sweet peas (frozen)

7. Asparagus
8. Honeydew melon
9. Kiwi
10. Cabbage
11. Watermelon
12. Mushrooms
13. Mangoes
14. Sweet potatoes
15. Carrots

PAN UK doesn't do a Clean Fifteen list. Why?

'PAN UK does not produce a so-called "Clean 15" list of produce with the least residues. This is because the government testing programme is so limited that we would not want to give the impression that certain produce is guaranteed to be free from pesticide cocktails. It is also possible to grow food using hazardous pesticides without the chemicals in question appearing as residues in food. As a result, an absence of residues should not be taken as assurance that there have been no pesticide-related harms to human health or the environment where the food was grown.'

This is why I wash or soak all my fruit and veg.

While there is significant overlap, the UK and US lists do differ slightly. This is due to differences in agricultural practices, pesticide regulations (a biggie), and the specific data used in the analysis. Overall, the Dirty Dozen and Clean Fifteen lists provide a great guide for us to make an informed choice about which fruits and vegetables to prioritise buying organic where possible.

Why am I so invested in this avoidance and removal of pesticides? Because pesticides are everywhere, especially, as you may have noted, in the 'healthier' foods, such as my favourites: celery, spinach and kale.

The significant use of pesticides was illuminated for me at a lecture on sustainable farming. Naively, I was unaware of how many chemicals many commercial farmers could be handling. I was blown away by the toxicity of the chemicals that are used and the impact that this, my further research revealed, would have on fertility.

Certain farming practices and agricultural chemicals have been found to negatively affect male fertility all over the world. The increase in general use of pesticides, herbicides and other substances commonly used in conventional farming can act as endocrine disruptors for men and women. Studies have linked exposure to these chemicals, often through handling. These chemicals used in farming have widely been reported to reduce sperm count, motility and quality in male farmers and farm workers. What does this mean for us the consumer, ingesting the contaminated produce?

The way we eat in the modern world has changed dramatically over the last few decades. No longer do we only have the option of locally produced foods, as we can go to the supermarket – or even local small greengrocers in the North of England – and get green beans from Kenya and strawberries out of season from Spain, Egypt, Morocco and Israel. We, as a population, have been fed (pardon the pun) the lie that bigger is better, and so farmers are producing larger produce. How do they do this? Also, how do the strawberries fly from Morocco to West Yorkshire and still not spoil? I know that on the occasion we have managed to grow the odd strawberry in our garden, and they don't last long.

Many farmers are under pressure to produce food at a lower price for the consumer, and pesticides can help increase yields. But, to my mind, this comes at a great cost. The cost of male and female reproductive health. Where we financially can, we need to support farmers who are adopting more sustainable, organic farming methods, not only for our health and their health and the health of their families, but also for the health of future generations.

Yes, of course, where you can, I would always encourage people to grow their own fruits and vegetables, but not all of us have the time or access to an allotment like my grandad did. Or maybe you are like me and your small garden doesn't have enough space to grow your own vegetables like my dad did in his garden. Or maybe you simply aren't green-fingered (also like me; in my family, I'm known as 'Doctor Death' when it comes to plants of any kind, even cactuses).

We have a very small garden and have tried to grow our own fruits and vegetables in plant pots. We managed some strawberries and courgettes, but our yield barely supported a family of three for one meal, never mind a week . . . However, there was such a difference in the taste, even to any organic produce I have ever bought. My little one is not a fan of courgette, but she gobbled these up in one go. As the flowers are edible, she had fun eating those too. One thing that has come back every year despite the harsh weather are the herbs, however, so that's one totally clean food source we can eat each week.

How to clean your fruits and veg that are not organic or homegrown.

Here are four effective methods to help reduce pesticide residues on fruits and vegetables:

1. Washing with vinegar solution
   Mix 1 part white vinegar with 3 parts water in a large bowl or sink.
   Soak the produce in the solution for 10–15 minutes, gently swishing it around.

Rinse thoroughly under running water.
This helps remove a significant amount of surface pesticides.
Best used with: apples, strawberries, leafy greens, potatoes.

2. Baking soda soak (this is what I do the most)
   Create a solution of 1 teaspoon baking soda per 2 cups of water.
   Soak the produce for 12–15 minutes, then rinse.
   Baking soda helps break down and remove pesticide residues.
   Best used with: grapes, blueberries, carrots, tomatoes.
   I would not advise this method with strawberries, as, in my experience, it spoils them.

3. Saltwater soak
   Mix 1 teaspoon of salt per 4 cups of water.
   Soak produce for 10–12 minutes and rinse thoroughly.
   The salt helps draw out and remove pesticides.
   Best used with: cucumbers, bell peppers, celery, peaches.

4. Scrubbing with a produce brush
   If you are old enough, like me, your parents or grandparents always used to do this. Somewhere along the way we have lost these best practices.

> Use a clean soft-bristle produce brush to gently scrub the surface of fruits and vegetables. This physically removes surface pesticides and dirt.

Now we have sorted how you prepare and cook your food, how do you clean the dishes, your clothes and your home?

On my own personal wellness journey, the small point of cleaning was one of the biggest challenges I faced when it came to cleaning up my life. However, after much trial and error, it also turned out to be one of the most cost-effective.

Cleaning the Kitchen

If you are reading this book and it's your sperm or your egg that's being used on your fertility journey, then in my mind 50% of your child-in-waiting is ready-made. So we need to be as gentle as we can with this delicate little egg and sperm that you're going to be using and we really don't want to blast them with harmful chemicals.

Just think, if you are inviting your favourite family member or best friend to a party at home, then you would want to give the house a good clean and make it as inviting for them as possible beforehand.

Here you are preparing for one of the most important birthdays in your life so far, the BIRTHday of your child.

So, how do we clean the dishes? The surfaces? The floor? Your clothes?

Washing up

Many of the popular washing-up liquids and dishwasher detergents that are most likely next to or under your sink, usually contain concerning chemicals that can disrupt your hormonal health. Ingredients like fragrances (you know about these now, but you may not have connected them to your washing-up liquid or dishwasher tablet), dyes and antimicrobial agents found in these cleaning products have been linked to hormone imbalances, fertility issues and other reproductive problems, along with skin issues and respiratory problems.

In 2023, a study from Switzerland shed new light on the concerning effects of alcohol ethoxylates, a common ingredient found in many dishwasher rinse aids. The findings were quite alarming. The researchers discovered that alcohol ethoxylates can disrupt the delicate balance of the gut microbiome, leading to a condition known as leaky gut.

The key messages from the data that they published were:

'Professional dishwasher rinse aid causes cellular cytotoxicity and directly impaired barrier integrity of gut epithelial cells by damaging TJ and AJ expressions in daily exposed concentrations.

'The underlying mechanisms of epithelial barrier disruption in response to rinse aid were cell death in 1:10,000 dilutions and epithelial barrier opening in 1:40,000 dilutions.

'The alcohol ethoxylates, an ingredient in the rinse aid that remains on washed dishware, caused the gut epithelial inflammation and barrier damage.'[47]

What does this mean in 'normal speak'?

Basically, even low-level residue left on our plates and dishes is harming us. These chemicals impair the integrity of the gut's epithelial barrier.

What's that, you ask?

The body is like your favourite house, where you want your guest to stay and thrive, be that the egg, the sperm or the embryo. Well, imagine this house has lots of different rooms, these are all the organs and body parts inside you. The kitchen (which in my mind is the hub of the home and where everyone congregates at a house party) would be your stomach, the living room would be your lungs, and so on.

Now, the epithelial barrier is kind of like the walls within that house. It's a special layer of cells that line the inside of your intestines, and it acts as a protective barrier. It's there to keep the good stuff, like the nutrients from your food, inside your body where they belong. But it also keeps the bad stuff, like germs or toxins, from getting in and making you sick.

You can think of the epithelial barrier as a really effective security guard for your body. The gatekeeper. It's always on the lookout, making sure nothing harmful gets past it and into your bloodstream. However, when certain chemicals or ingredients damage or weaken this epithelial barrier, it's like the security guard is injured and can no longer do their job properly. This is when you can start to have problems like your gut getting inflamed or your body not being able to absorb nutrients as well. You feel sluggish, have brain fog, headaches, all sorts of things.

When the gut barrier is compromised in this way, it allows undigested food particles, toxins (this nasty rinse-aid chemical, for example) and bacteria to 'leak' through into the bloodstream. This then triggers an inflammatory immune response, and inflammation has been linked to a range of chronic health issues, including autoimmune disorders, food allergies and digestive problems.[48] Leaky gut is something I have had, and it makes you feel awful, trust me. It's something you want to avoid, or if you think you have it, take steps to repair it, not only for your fertility journey but your overall health.

We need optimal digestion so we can absorb and use all the nutrients from our food, and we want to reduce inflammation, which can negatively affect conception, sperm results and implantation.

The good news is that there are now more natural, plant-derived alternatives available for dishwasher rinse aids and dishwasher cleaning products. You can even get plant-derived sheets that you can dissolve for hand-washing dishes in the sink. I encourage you to carefully read product labels and seek out plant-derived rinse aid options next time you need to restock your dishwashing supplies, because, as you now see, it's not just what's on your plate that can feed or disrupt the gut, but the plate itself.

Even the seemingly more 'natural' dishwasher tablets can contain hormone-disrupting substances like phosphates and chlorine. So do check what the product is made of and don't just look at the label; check out the brand's website and find the full ingredients and fact sheets. Once again, it seems the smaller brands are the leading champions when it comes to making these changes.

What to be on the lookout for that may be chemicals for concern:

Fragrances – can disrupt hormones, cause allergic reactions and affect your thyroid. I for one get very dizzy and nauseous when exposed to strong chemical fragrances in cleaning products. Even many that say they are 'eco' can have chemical fragrances in them.

Dyes – linked to hormone imbalances and reproductive issues.

Phosphates – endocrine disruptors that can impact fertility.

Chlorine – a harsh chemical that can mimic oestrogen in the body.

Antimicrobial agents (like triclosan) – shown to interfere with thyroid function.

Plastics in the dishwasher tablets: The high heat and intense scrubbing action of the dishwasher can cause plastics to break down and leach chemicals onto the dishes. This is particularly problematic for plastics like polycarbonate, which contains the hormone-disrupting chemical bisphenol A (BPA). Even 'BPA-free' plastics may contain other bisphenol compounds that can also interfere with endocrine function.

The melting and degradation of plastic crockery in the dishwasher allows these chemicals to seep into your food, leading to ongoing exposure and potential hormonal havoc. It's best to avoid washing plastic containers, cups and utensils in the dishwasher when possible, and opt for glass, ceramic or stainless-steel alternatives instead.

Once again, I'm not here to scaremonger, but to inform and educate you so you can slowly do you own research and try out a few cleaner brands. Once you have found a good one, all the hard work is done. You can even make your own. I don't always have time to (with writing this book, sometimes I don't even have time to shower!), but here are some great recipes.

Making your own non-toxic dishwasher cleaner and rinse aid is actually quite simple! Here are some easy eco-friendly recipes you can try at home.

Note: Certain essential oils are not good for pets, so do bear this in mind.

Dishwasher cleaner

- 1 cup baking soda
- ½ cup washing soda/soda crystals (not to be confused with baking soda) or ½ cup citric acid powder
- 10–15 drops of lemon or orange essential oil (optional for scent)

Mix the baking soda and washing soda together in a jar or container. Add the essential oil if you want a fresh, citrusy smell.

Use 1–2 tablespoons of this homemade powder in each dishwasher load, adding it to the tablet area. The baking soda and washing soda will gently clean and deodorise your dishes without any harsh chemicals.

Dishwasher rinse aid

1 cup white vinegar
10–15 drops of lemon or lavender essential oil (optional)

Pour the vinegar into a clean spray bottle and add the essential oil drops if desired. Shake to combine. After your dishwasher cycle is complete, simply spray this rinse aid solution onto your clean dishes. The vinegar helps remove any remaining food particles and water spots, leaving your dishes sparkling clean.

Cleaning the surfaces

It makes sense that what we spray in our homes gets not only onto the surfaces but also our food, our skin and most certainly into the air. As I've said, often the biggest culprits are the chemical fragrances and dyes. Brands know what they are doing when they make their products bright colours and make them smell of forests or summer days spent in a flower-filled garden. They are appealing to our senses.

Next, think of thyroid-disrupting bleach, especially in bathroom cleaner. We've all used those harsh brands where even after the first two sprays you start coughing and have to open the door and windows. Many years ago, I did a deep clean on a rental I was leaving. I had my cleaning gloves on, but before I had finished the first bathroom, the gloves had started to disintegrate, and my hands had become red raw. By bathroom two they had started to bleed. If I was using similar chemicals in my kitchen daily and then chopping vegetables for dinner for my family, what effect would these chemicals be having on me and my family?

I did a deep dive into this topic, and it wasn't pleasant reading. There were many links to both breast cancer and uterine cancer. I didn't want to put them in the book because we don't need scaring any more, but just knowing that those studies exist, for me, is enough to find an alternative. I really would encourage you to choose natural cleaners without chemical fragrances or bleach, because the standards in the UK mean that not all ingredients have to be listed, even on 'eco' products. For example, your chosen brand may state 'fragrance' on the label, but we don't know what that fragrance is made from. Also, don't forget many cleaning products are in plastic containers, and we all know plastics are not great for us.

If you want to make your own cleaning products, here are some kitchen and bathroom cleaning recipes.

Kitchen cleaner

Vinegar and Water Cleaner
Mix 1 part white vinegar with 1 part water in a glass spray bottle.

This is a simple solution that effectively cuts through grease and grime on countertops, sinks and other kitchen surfaces.

Baking soda and Castile soap cleaner
In a glass spray bottle, combine 2 cups water, ¼ cup baking soda and 2 tablespoons liquid Castile soap. Shake well before each use.

This all-purpose cleaner is great for cleaning surfaces and good for wooden chopping boards.

What is Castile soap, you may ask? Castile soap is a type of soap made from 100% vegetable oils, without any animal fats or synthetic detergents. Castile soap is traditionally made from olive oil, though some modern versions may use a blend of vegetable oils, olive oil and coconut oil. It's also great for a body wash. Plus, it does not contain any animal products, so it's vegan friendly. Here the baking soda provides gentle abrasion while the Castile soap helps lift dirt.

Lemon and Castile soap cleaner
Mix 1 cup water, ¼ cup lemon juice, and 1 tablespoon Castile soap in a glass spray bottle. Shake to combine. The citric acid in lemon juice helps deodorise and cut through grease, while the Castile soap provides cleaning power.

Oven cleaner

Baking soda and vinegar (the one I do fortnightly)
Sprinkle baking soda generously over the interior of the oven, including the racks. Spray or pour white vinegar over the baking soda. It will create a foaming reaction. Let the mixture sit for 15–20 minutes to break down grease and grime. Wipe clean with a damp cloth or sponge.

Lemon juice and salt
Make a paste with lemon juice and table salt. Spread the paste over the interior of the oven. Let the mixture sit for 15–20 minutes, then wipe clean.

The acidity in the lemon helps cut through baked-on grime, plus it then smells pretty too.

Castile soap and water
Mix a few drops of unscented Castile soap with warm water. Use a sponge or cloth to scrub the oven walls and racks. Wipe clean with a damp cloth.

Steam cleaning
Place a baking dish filled with water in the oven, add the lemon juice from half a lemon and run a self-cleaning cycle. The steam will help loosen built-up grime for easier wiping.

Bathroom cleaner

Tea Tree

1 cup white vinegar
10 drops eucalyptus essential oil
10 drops tea tree essential oil
¼ cup baking soda

Mix the vinegar, eucalyptus and tea tree oils in a glass spray bottle. Add the baking soda and shake to combine. Spray on surfaces and wipe clean.

You could even add a sprig of rosemary. You would need to change it every few days, but it looks pretty in the bathroom and smells delightful.

Frankincense bathroom scrub

This is the first one I made after I had the run-in with the bleach cleaner that made my hands bleed when I was sick with lupus.

1 cup baking soda
10 drops frankincense essential oil
Water as needed

Mix the baking soda and frankincense in a bowl.

Add water a little at a time until it forms a thick paste. Gently scrub onto surfaces and let sit for a few minutes before wiping clean.

Cleaning clothes

Vinegar and baking soda detergent

1 cup baking soda
1 cup washing soda
1 cup Castile soap or liquid soap
20–30 drops essential oils (optional)

Mix the baking soda and washing soda.
Add the liquid soap and essential oils (if using).
Use 1–2 tablespoons per load.
Add ½ cup white vinegar to the rinse cycle for softening.

If you are old enough, you may recall your grandparents using these sorts of recipes. I remember my dad using newspaper and vinegar to do the windows and beeswax to polish the wood in the house. So many of these replacements don't have to cost a lot of money, and more than likely the homemade versions will be much cheaper to make than even your low-cost own-brand cleaners in the supermarkets.

These also make for great gifts and you can personalise them with your friends' or family members' favourite essential oils.

Week 9. Investing in Self. Investing in the Couple. Making Love, Not a Baby

Let's talk about sex, baby. Vitamin L. Love and lust. The best and most over-looked vitamin in the world when it comes to any type of health and wellbeing.

One of the many topics that come up when I'm coaching couples on the road to parenthood is not only the loss of intimacy around sex, but many men especially say all the romance and spontaneity has gone out of the relationship and they feel that trying to conceive has taken over the relationship.

It certainly can take over the finances. Holidays have had to be forsaken, buying a home put on hold, loans may have been taken out, extra workload taken on to pay for it all, and the finances are simply stretched to their limits. And so is the mind from juggling all the numbers.

People start to feel invisible to their partner, and couples can become emotionally detached from one another. Particularly when the only topic of conversation is fertility. Or the lack of.

That 'infertility' has become their label, their macrocosm, their world. It is monopolising their bank account, lifestyle, mind, conversations and even their sex life. And stress is on the rise. Stress is a big endocrine disruptor. A sniper for the libido. When people turn around to couples struggling with infertility and say, 'Oh, I bet you are having fun trying, though,' they clearly have not been in your shoes, as that ovulation window can be anything but fun. Hence why I like to bring some fun and romance back in. Let's release some of those wonderful happy hormones and take the pressure off during what is a very pressurised time.

1. In the words of Justin Timberlake, 'Bring sexy back.'

Remember back to when you had sex for sex's sake? Can you? People often tell a couple struggling with fertility to 'Just relax', or 'Go on holiday, it will happen.' Ha, these people just don't know, do they?

Day in, day out I see couples where sex for sex's sake has been taken off the menu, period. Apart from four circled dates on an app, it does not happen. I have women tell me they tell their partners to 'hurry up', as they need to get to sleep, or couples setting the alarm an hour earlier so they can get 'it' done before work.

Sex has become a chore. Just as the bins need taking out or the dishwasher needs emptying . . .

This kind of sex to make a baby does not help your relationship with each other or your relationship to yourself. If you're having intercourse and feeling stressed about it, dreading it, feeling like it's merely a perfunctory action, it is neither good for your relationship nor good for your body.

In some cases, sex becomes a crisis. Men feel the pressure so much that they end up abandoning the sex because they can't get an erection at the right time. I've had male clients secretly taking Viagra or asking me for an extra private session where they talk in the car about how they feel pressured, used and unattractive. Sex is no longer about them as a person, just about trying to make a baby.

Unfortunately, not many men feel that they can turn to their friends, because guys in general don't talk about infertility. With unhelpful friends likely making jokes, saying they must be 'firing blanks', or a 'stiff drink will get them going' or even 'I can lend a hand.' Plus, some feel that they can't talk to their partner because they don't want to stress them out even more. If you feel like this, you are not alone, and this week's exercises will help bring it up in conversation and give you some fun tools to address it.

It's not just the chaps. All too often I see women who feel like their body is failing them. That through all the trials and tribulations of fertility, they have become almost detached from their own femininity. They no longer feel that physiological sexual urge leading up to ovulation because it's become a mental strategic marathon instead.

So many people are working even longer hours and often bring work home with them, and added to that, there are continuously pinging WhatsApp groups and social media apps to check . . . our information overload is monumental nowadays. The last thing most of us want to do when we finally get to stop at night is have sex because our fertility app says GO AT IT NOW!

Do you remember the days when sex had nothing to do with making a baby, nothing to do with waiting for a missed period?

News flash! Sex is not just for ovulation. Bring sex back in all its forms for the rest of the month together.

Court each other, flirt, engage in foreplay, try to make your partner feel special and sexy. They are not a machine or a chore to be 'done'. Keep the TV out of the bedroom, and phones too (if you need the phone for an alarm, place it near your bedroom door – or get an alarm clock). In the evening, go back to pillow talk, play cards, or, dare I say it, TALK to each other!

I don't care if you are working from home and the cleaner is there (remember when you were in your twenties? Like this sort of thing would have stopped you . . . it may even have excited you).

I get it, many of us have long commutes, work long hours, some have children to look after, we get tired. It doesn't have to be a sex Olympics, nor does it have to be full penetration. In the time outside of ovulation, shine a spotlight on oral sex, for example. It can be using your hands, fingers. Your partner doesn't even have to be there; bring on the masturbation. Self-pleasure is a great tool to connect you to your body. Touch yourself, remember what it feels like to feel sexy and sensual when, especially for females, you may feel that your body has become a means of fertility only. Many clients going through IVF say that they feel their body is no longer their own. This is a time to reconnect.

I love supplements. I love removing and replacing common things in my clients' lives. But I have yet to find anything that comes close to the benefits of a good orgasm. When we reach a climax and experience an orgasm, we release amazing hormones that target inflammation and that make you feel good about yourself during what can be, for some, an immensely stressful time. You may not have been sleeping well because you're worried about the rising costs of fertility treatment, there is a baby shower to attend, your friend got pregnant yet she eats rubbish, and though you are happy for her you can't help but feel it's not fair . . . It's a trying time. Take yourself for a 10-minute masturbation session, have an orgasm, and it will literally change your brain. You'll release a flood of oxytocin, or the 'love hormone', and dopamine, the 'feel-good' neurotransmitter. It's a boost of nourishment, and it's free! It's a great tool for taking the edge off, especially now alcohol is off the table, as could be your favourite go-to sweet treat in times of stress.

Plus, the more we stimulate the sexual organs, the more we want it. Therefore, the more we include masturbation or cunnilingus or the odd blow job or hand job, the more as a couple you will want sex throughout the month and not just in that blue window or when the ovulation sticks demand or temperature checks suggest.

Consider buying a book on sex. There is so much to learn. We often go with what we know, but did you know there are erogenous zones all over the body, not just the genitalia or neck and ears, but on the calf and knee, for example?

Learning a new sexual skill, massage, sexy toys, all make intercourse about something more than procreation.

Don't focus on the penetration either.

Sex for women, I find often starts earlier in the day, earlier in the week. Those pecks on the cheek, a kiss when greeted at the door. (Oh, wait a minute, actually go greet your partner at the door, instead of waiting until they walk in the room and you look up from whatever digital device you are glued to and grunt some form of recognition.)

We often leave these all-important acts of affection behind in the later years of relationships. Then we have the cheek to complain that sex is not what it was. Ask yourself what else is different now from the start of the relationship. What can you realistically bring back?

Here are some homework activities to bring romance back:

Mission one: The £10 date

'Just relax and the baby will come.' This was the most fire-fuelling, stressful advice anyone gave me when I was trying for another child. But they were right. Distractions and fun will help lessen what at times can be an all-consuming topic. Ovulation sticks, temperature checks, sex on certain days, changes in habits, medical investigations, navigating everyone else's pregnancies. Why is it that when you are trying to get pregnant, your friends, the woman down the road, celebrities, your friend's friend, people after one-night stands, in movies, everyone is doing it and getting success, but not you?

Here is where the £10 date can create some much-needed frivolity, creativity and fun.

Each week, or biweekly, depending on your available free time, it will be the responsibility of one person in the couple to create a £10 date for you both to go on. Or, if you are single, you do it for yourself. The only rule is that ALL the £10 must be spent. Why I love the £10 date is because it forces you to be creative.

Some great examples from clients are:

(Steal them if you want, no one will know!)

'My mate needs a man with a van.'

One gentleman borrowed a white minivan and a projector under the ruse that he 'needed to move something for a friend' and he needed his wife's help to do so, as the 'friend' would be out. He then drove 30 minutes in no particular direction, parked up and showed her what was waiting in the back. Cushions, blankets, a movie they watched on one of their first dates, and a picnic. This was the foreplay they both needed. It wasn't a flash meal where you eat so much the last thing you want to do when you go home is have sex, as you are stuffed to the brim. It wasn't a spa for a weekend, where you are surrounded by other couples or under the gaze of hen dos. It was good old-fashioned romance and spontaneity.

Next time I see a little white van parked up and no one is in the driver's seat, I hope you are in the back making happy memories.

'Cabin the woods, or at the end of your parents' garden.'

Another couple were living with the husband's parents while their house was undergoing a roof repair. They were finding this lack of privacy and added financial pressure an added stress to their fertility journey and were coping by BOTH going to work early and coming home late. The wife decided to take the afternoon off and decorate the hut at the end of the parents' garden with fairy lights and tea lights and recreated one of their first date meals.

When the husband came in, he cried. She'd only spent £8 and donated the remaining £2. Sex on a picnic blanket at the end of your parents' garden is something you do in your younger years when you are free and full of hormones. This dopamine rush and connection is what we most need; a break from timed sex just because the app says so.

'Cheese, please.'

My partner and I regularly did the £10 challenge on our fertility journey while living in London, and one of my favourite £10 dates was when he took me to a cheese museum. It was really a cheese shop, but you could go out the back and see how it was all made and they would talk you through the cheeses, and, boy, do we both love cheese!

To save the money for the cheese, we had to walk there and back, which ended up as a three-hour round trip. This gifted us the added bonus of seeing London as tourists, something we had not done in our twenty-plus years living and working in the city, often too busy getting to where we were going to see where we were. My tip in any city is look up. I still go to London and look up and see new things all the time.

Mission two: Recreate your second date

The second date is often the day that you decide, 'I really like this person.' You start to let your barriers down. You make a huge effort. I recall my second date with my partner. We went to the Victoria and Albert Museum, which was having an exhibition on lingerie through the ages. And after, as we walked and walked around in the late summer night, we devised a magical mystery tour. Each of us would choose a direction, straight on, left or right, into unknown streets until we came across the second (as it was our second date) restaurant, where we would eat. You could drive to a local town or village and do the same thing.

Spontaneity, the unknown, creates memories, but also taking an element from your joyful memory bank will really let your partner know that they are seen because, quite often on the fertility journey, the recognition of the individual can be lost or become faded. This bond is so important to work on as you start and continue on your fertility journey.

Mission three: Don't change your dreams or your calendar

You are still you. Your fertility journey does NOT define you. You don't need to stay in and be a hermit because you are not drinking alcohol. You can still go to the pub, to the bar, go out with family for your Sunday dinner, simply remove and replace and make different choices. The show must go on.

Don't try and map out the future with 'what ifs'. 'We can't book that holiday because what if I'm pregnant then', 'We won't want to have the kitchen redone if we have a newborn.' To my mind the baby will come when it comes and will slot in just fine. The baby doesn't care if your kitchen is being done, if it's on a plane, at a wedding. It just wants love, a cuddle and milk. And guess what, it doesn't know any different.

Mission four: No-fertility-talk days

According to the Society of Assisted Reproductive Technology, undergoing fertility treatment is as stressful, if not more stressful, than a number of key life events, including the death of a family member. A Fertility Network UK survey found that '59% reported some detrimental impact of fertility problems and/or treatment on the relationship with their partner.'

Yes, you have this book, yes, you are trying for a baby or thinking of trying for a baby in the future or have tried and are having a break, or maybe you're just about to embark on your first or fifth round of IVF, but take a break from talking about it as a couple. I like to give my clients 'no TTC' (trying to conceive) talk days. Just as you have an ovulation window where sex is under the spotlight, have a couples window, where you focus conversations on you as a couple. All your other dreams deserve space too.

Mission five: Sex ban in the bedroom

Last, but certainly not least, sex in the bedroom at the end of the night is banned! You can have sex (and I highly recommend it as a first step to fertility – he he!) but it has to be any place but the bedroom and never at the end of the night.

There's nothing like sex when you come home from work, to leave the day job behind and cleanse the soul for the rest of the evening. My male clients always light up when I introduce this little slice of homework. They often go from being a glazed-over slumped figure on the Zoom meeting to almost standing to attention (pardon the pun) and being Mr Perky Chappy, all wide-eyed with glee. The week after, I might add, the female client is also wide-eyed with glee. This week is going to be a good week!

I love you, body, I'm sorry, let's make friends (for the ladies)

When I ask women at the initial consultation why they have chosen to get in touch now, they often say because they feel they've lost themselves to IVF, and they can't do another round of IVF mentally or physically, and they need help to get stronger. They want to feel like themselves again because of late they have felt that their body, hormones and their mind are now in the hands of the IVF doctors. Or they've tried naturally for a year with no progress.

In reply to this, I always ask them the same questions.

How do you feel towards your body? What would you say to it if it could hear? What do you secretly say to it in your head?

They often reply with the following:

'I feel betrayed.'

'I'm disappointed in it.'

'I feel like it's/I'm a failure.'

'I feel like it's let me down.'

'I feel like my body is no longer my own.'

'I no longer feel feminine.'

'I'm angry at my body.'

'I hate my body.'

'I feel numb.'

'I feel no connection to my body.'

'I wonder what I did wrong.'

I understand all these emotions; I too battled with them when I was struggling with my fertility. So it is not my aim to judge here, but rather to release the negativity held within.

The book *The Body Keeps the Score* by renowned psychiatrist Bessel van der Kolk[49] explores how trauma impacts the mind and body, and I believe that an infertility diagnosis for many, women especially, is a trauma. I believe that when we're holding such anger, sadness, contempt and frustration, it can create a tightness in the body that can lead to inflammation as well as an imbalance in the gut and hormones. When the body is stressed, even if it's silent stress or holding on to anger, it is less able to digest its food, absorb all the nutrients from the nutrient-dense food that we're consuming and absorb the vitamins and minerals we are supplementing the body with.

I truly believe that the body listens to all that we say, even in our silence. So start to listen to the conversation that you are having with it. Is it one of kindness? Again, no judgement, I simply want you to listen in to the words you use around your fertility journey, and also the unspoken words that go around in your head.

> 'Throughout the TTC process, I'd forgotten how to have sex just for fun, my mind was consumed with ovulation and timings. This session really focused on bringing sexy back and made me feel better about myself also remembering what turns us on as a couple, which created that excitement and those loving feelings we had prior to the journey. Loved it.'
>
> Chantelle

Week 10. Diet

The word 'diet' has become, to my mind, very negative. With connotations of restriction, it brings up feelings of deprivation, something you do short term almost as a punishment.

No.

I prefer the true meaning of the word diet. Let's look at its origins. The word diet comes from the Greek δίαιτα (*diaita*), which represents a notion of a whole 'way of living'. In fact, *diaita* is derived from the verb *diaitas*, meaning 'to lead one's life'. A true healthy way of living includes nurturing both mental and physical health, rather than a restrictive short-term weight-loss regimen.

As you will grasp by now, 'diet' isn't just the food you put on your plate. Yet that is how we have become accustomed to thinking about it.

I prefer to see it as an 'inclusion' rather than an 'exclusion'. Diet is about what we can invest in and gain rewards from in all aspects of our lives rather than what we are abstaining from.

As we are in the world of slogans, I may as well start off with two.

'You are what you eat.'

'You are what you eat has eaten.'

The latter one not many people think about, but it's true nonetheless.

I often say to clients when they first come to me with their food diary, not in a mean way but a genuine question: 'Would you feed your child-in-waiting this diet?' and 'Would you expect your child to thrive if you gave them this diet?'

More often than not, people say, 'No, I would not give this to my child.'

Some common responses:

'There is way too much junk.'

'There's too much sugar.'

'There's not enough protein.'

'There's not enough variety, I eat the same lunch every day.'

'I only really eat one meal a day, no wonder I'm always starving in the evening.'

'I snack late in the evening because I'm hungry, because I don't feed myself during the day, but I will treat my child better.'

You are what you eat has eaten

Bear with me as I'm going to tell you a little story about my eggs. Not the ones in my ovaries, but the ones with which I often make a courgette, asparagus and coconut-flour omelette for my lunch.

Today, to take my mandatory break from the laptop, I went for a little walk to one of the farms up near where I live to buy some eggs. And the reason I go to this farm and not to the local supermarket, or even buy the organic ones in the big supermarket, is because of three things. In no particular order:

1. I want to support the local community.
2. They have a sign outside that says, 'I only feed them the best things. P.S. They are spoilt rotten.'
3. If I continue walking up the lane and around the field, I can see the 'spoilt rotten' hens running around having

the best time. And we all know that when we humans eat healthy food and run around, aka exercise, we feel great. We're outdoors with good light and fresh air in the elements. When we live like this, our body thanks us for it. That's why I go and buy my eggs there and sometimes I even leave a little extra as a tip. I want the best-quality eggs inside me and that goes for your eggs too. For me, it's the ones in my omelette and for you ladies it's the ones in your omelette and the ones inside your ovaries.

And I want you, whether woman or a man, to start thinking about the quality and variety of your food. As I mentioned before, I prefer to focus on what we put in, rather than what we abstain from. And that's also how this farmer invests in her livestock. She puts in the love, the commitment, the feed, the space, so the hens can produce such fine eggs. I know not everyone has a farm around the corner, or a local house with a few hens, but many of us can start asking where our food is from. Maybe you'll even buy a hen or two yourselves?

I encourage you to invest in your food, because you're not just feeding yourself. Just like a mummy who is pregnant, and who is feeding her baby, you are now also feeding your eggs or sperm.

Yes, I'm also going to say what not to eat, but as far as I'm concerned, this isn't even food, so I'm not asking you to be restrictive in your diet!

I would be remiss if I did not address UPF (ultra-processed foods). Finally UPFs are getting the bad press they deserve.

I know you know the score on this, even before I go ahead and say what I have to say. It's simply not even food as far as I'm concerned, so let's call these mainly chemical formulations 'digestibles'.

Treat/Cheat Day

Oh my gosh, if there is one phrase from some PTs that gets my goat, it's 'treat day' or 'cheat day'. Trust me, you are treating yourself when you eat all that nature has given us. When you eat as close to the Mediterranean diet as possible. When you cook from scratch. When you get back to basics. This is the best treat you can give your body, your mind, your future self and your child-in-waiting. I think 'cheat day' is more honest and on point, because you are cheating yourself, your future self and your future goals and all the work you have already done. Rant over.

So, bin the phrase and bin the practice and bin the mindset.

Often a cheat day means some form of takeaway.

Here are just some of the issues with most takeaways available and how they sabotage your fertility fitness. (Takeaway hot drinks are also included here, unless they're in your own portable cup.)

Most takeaways come in some kind of plastic container. (Do you remember the chapter on plastics and endocrine disruptors?) The EWG (Environmental Working Group) stated in 2024 that 'Research shows adults take in up to 150,000 plastic particles annually via their diet.'[50] They estimate that this is the equivalent to consuming up to twelve plastic shopping bags per year. With recent research finding plastic particles in human tissue and even placenta, it's time to rethink 'cheat day' and 'treat day'. If this doesn't put you off your Friday night chicken kebab and chips or your takeaway latte, I don't know what will.

Inflammatory oils cooked at a high heat, and most likely in a toxic non-stick pan, are not going to be your fertile friend.

Takeaway companies need to make a profit and will do so more often than not by sourcing the cheapest low-grade ingredients. It makes economical sense, but not fertility sense.

There is no point splashing your cash on supplements, no

point in going to the gym (you will never exercise your way out of a bad diet), if you continue to have cheat days. They will never serve your higher needs.

I recently had a couple who were eating two or three takeaways a week as some kind of pat on the back for starting the gym and taking all their supplements. These were two very highly educated people. They had degrees coming out of their ears and more letters after their name than I will ever have, so they knew full well it was not serving their goal. But like many people, they were addicted to the dopamine hit, not only from the food, but from believing they were giving themselves a treat. And, yes, I do believe they were addicted.

My job as their coach was to not only change their mindset, but also to slowly wean them off their takeaways with a dopamine-hit replacement to prevent them having an almighty setback and kicking everything to the kerb, including me.

I likened their takeaway 'treats' to a gambling addict just popping to the casino for one game of roulette. The casino is the shop or food-delivery service, the game is your chosen UPF. Roulette is a super-quick game and most certainly gets your dopamine firing through the roof. Only, just as quickly as that ball spins around the wheel, when it DOES NOT fall on your colour, the crash happens, and that's why for most people, especially an addict, it's never just one game of roulette, is it? Just as it's never just one square of chocolate or one bite of cake ... The gambling addict also doesn't just go to the casino once or open their gambling app just a few times a month. No, for some it's every day or in the evenings after work or at the weekend as a treat because they've been 'good' all week. They say there is only one winner in the casino, and that is the casino, not the player. I think it's just the same with ultra-processed food. You think you are winning when you take those first few tasty mouthfuls, but really it's taking you further and further away from your goals and distancing you from your 'why'.

This was the advice I gave that couple and now I give it to you with the same heart. Have a read and then we can crack on and look at some great REAL foods to play with.

1. I want you to start parenting yourselves and replace the takeouts with a detailed food plan for breakfast, lunch, dinner, snacks. (I will give you a sample one – one vegetarian, one flexitarian – it's not a rule, rather a guide. I want you to start experimenting and building a beautiful relationship with food.) There's no point fasting at breakfast, and having a tiny salad or a meal replacement shake for lunch and a handful of nuts, if, by the time you get home, you feel burnt out and can't sleep. Then, by the time you get halfway through the week, you need a takeaway and more treats. Then the next day you feel

you failed with the takeaway so you may as well have a piece of cake, a cookie, a beer. I mean, after all, you didn't eat till midday, did you?

2. Replace the late-night dopamine hit from takeaways with natural dopamine hits that don't lead to such a crash, slump, dump, that don't raise your inflammation, trash your sleep and your gut, and make your hormones feel like they are playing musical bumps on high speed. If you remove anything from your diet, it's important to replace it with something else. You are then much more likely to stick to it. So, take an evening walk instead of slumping in front of the TV or doomscrolling, as activity is great for regulating blood sugars after a meal. Perhaps replicate your favourite takeaway dish or banquet with a homemade Indian, burger or Chinese, then raise those happy hormones with an evening kitchen disco. When the sugar cravings come, instead of reaching for the packaged UPFs, create a decorative fruit platter; yes, fruit has sugar, but it's unrefined sugar and balanced with natural waters and fibre that will help regulate blood sugar spikes.

3. If, like me, you work from home, rather than rooting around in the fridge or the freezer on your breaks, go do some laps around the garden. If you have only a few minutes while the kettle boils, drop to the floor and do some sit-ups, star jumps or jump lunges (these get you going for sure). I just did some grounding in the garden.

I took off my shoes and socks and stood in the wet grass for 5 minutes to recharge myself. I also turned my face to the sun before I came back to my computer. You could even just jump up and down and do some shaking and patting the body; it will serve your body better than a can of something fizzy and a biscuit. It's about exploring things that bring your energy up and give you that dopamine hit that you have been so conditioned to receive.

Eat the Rainbow

As the saying goes, 'Variety is the spice of life', and it's also the key to thriving too.

There are seven colours in the rainbow. These are red, orange, yellow, green, blue, indigo and violet. Note, none of them are beige!

Red foods

Tomatoes: Tomatoes are fabulous for male fertility, as they contain lycopene, which has been proven to boost sperm quality.

Cherries: Cherries can benefit female fertility by providing antioxidants that may help reduce inflammation and support egg health. They are great to eat on your bleed too if you are prone to menstrual cramps.

Watermelon: Watermelon is known as natures Viagra. It contains citrulline, which is an amino acid that not only benefits circulation but may help improve erectile disfunction.

Raspberries: Raspberries are high in both vitamin C and folate, so they're great for both female and male fertility.

Pomegranate: One cup of pomegranate gives around 20% of your daily recommended amount of vitamin C, over 30% of your daily recommended amount of copper and around 17% of your daily recommended amount of folate.

Red lentils: Red lentils are a low-cost food that can be used in curries, as a replacement for rice, made into a mash or even as a porridge. They are abundant in protein, iron and B6.

Orange foods (orange for ovulation)

Citrus foods: If you slice an orange, lemon, lime or grapefruit open, to me it resembles not only the ovaries but also the vagina. Nature leaves clues for what to eat for what, and this is a big sign! Ever noticed that walnuts look like a brain? They are amazing for brain health!

Pumpkin: Not only is the flesh of a pumpkin full of nutrients for fertility, but the seeds are also abundant in zinc, so they're great to snack on for sperm health.

Sweet potato: One cup gives you 40% of your daily recommended amount of vitamin C and 15% of your daily recommended amount of potassium.

Yellow foods

Butternut squash: Butternut squash is low in calories and high in nutrients. One cup of cooked butternut squash will give you 400% of your daily recommended amount of vitamin A and contribute 7g of fibre. In the UK the recommended daily amount of fibre is around 30g for an adult.

Chickpeas: Low cost and super versatile, one cup of the humble chickpea gives you over 30% of your daily recommend amount of protein. They're also full of fibre and B vitamins.

Green foods

Broccoli: Broccoli is great for male and female fertility, as it contains about 90% of our daily recommended amount of vitamin C per cup.

Fresh parsley: Parsley is a great way to build your iron, especially if you don't eat red meat. One cup of fresh parsley equates to just over 20% of your daily recommended amount of iron.

Asparagus: Asparagus is beneficial for male and female fertility because it is rich in folate, providing approximately 34% of the daily recommended amount per cup.

Blue foods

Think of the blue sea here, so lots of fish for omega-3 and protein.

Purple/(indigo and violet) foods

Figs: Figs are supportive of male fertility especially, as they are rich in minerals like zinc and magnesium.

Plums: Remember, fruits with a P make you poo! Plums are high in fibre and water, so they're great for the detoxification process as well as hydration.

Blueberries: Blueberries were one of the first foods to be given the trendy label of 'superfood', and for good reason, as they are packed with antioxidants.

Purple sweet potato: Not only is the purple sweet potato full of antioxidants, it's also packed with vitamin C, manganese and copper. Half a cup of this root veg, once baked, will give you over 200% of your daily recommended amount of vitamin A. Vitamin A plays a vital role in sperm and egg development, but it is also crucial for placental health, foetal tissue development and foetal growth.

Red cabbage: Another low-cost food that is packed full of Vitamin C.

Beetroot: Beetroot looks like blood and that's what it helps – it's great for blood flow. It's also high in calcium, iron and folate.

Omega-3

The quality of your omega-3 is just as important as the quantity.

To ensure you're getting the best, opt for clean fatty fish, like salmon (wild, not farmed), mackerel, herring, kippers, pilchards, sardines and trout. (Not everyone is a fan of fish, so this is where your supplements come in handy.)

These fishes are not only rich in omega-3 but are also less likely to be contaminated with harmful pollutants and heavy metals. White fish is brilliant as well, especially haddock, as it's a great source of iodine. Iodine supports the thyroid and is important not only for women trying to conceive, but also once pregnant. It's important to keep those iodine levels balanced.

Oils

Pay attention to the oils you choose to cook with and also how you cook with them.

Good-quality oils, such as cold-pressed extra virgin olive oil, flaxseed oil or avocado oil, can provide a reliable source of omega-3.

Avoid oils that are heavily processed or contain additives, such as sunflower oil, rapeseed oil, palm oil or mixed vegetable oil.

I prefer, when medium frying, to use ghee or organic coconut oil, but mostly I will boil or steam and add oil afterwards.

Ghee has been in my life for about fifteen years now. I like it because it has a high smoking point, even higher than butter. It does have quite a distinct flavour, so you might not want to use it in baking, etc., but you can add it to your coffee or porridge, as it gives a beautiful buttery richness to the oats, which is wonderfully grounding in the colder months. Ghee is great for fertility, as it is rich in vitamins A, D, E and K, plus it's great for the gut too.

Folate

The food sources listed here are very low-cost as well as cross-seasonal, bar the asparagus.

> Asparagus
> Black beans
> Dark leafy greens
> Lentils
> Liver (higher in protein and iron than chicken breast and often much cheaper)
> Nuts
> Pinto beans
> Spinach

Protein

It doesn't matter if you are vegan, vegetarian, pescatarian or flexitarian. With food planning and weekly food prep, you can make sure you maintain your protein levels.

> Beans
> Lean meats
> Lentils

Nuts
Oats
Oily fish
Pulses
White fish (low on the mercury scale)

Fats

Avocado
Coconut oil
Eggs
Ghee
Nuts
Oily fish
Seeds, e.g. flaxseeds

B vitamin foods

Bananas
Broccoli
Fish (low on mercury scale)
Liver
Meat (grass-fed, organic, or the best you can realistically afford)

Nuts
Organic dairy
Oysters
Sweet potato
Whole grains

Hydrating foods

Apples
Broccoli
Celery
Cucumber
Dark purple berries
Green beans
Kale
Pineapple
Spinach
Watermelon

Gut foods – prebiotic and probiotic foods
(Think: G for gifts to my body)

Asparagus
Avocado

Cacao
Chicory root
Flaxseed
Kefir
Kimchi
Leeks
Oats
Sauerkraut

Fertility foods to rotate

Avocado
Bone broth
Dark berries
Dark leafy greens
Eggs
Gluten-free oats
Grass-fed meat (small portion)
Lentils
Oily fish
Organic full-fat Greek yoghurt
Pomegranate
Radish
Seafood
Sweet potato

Bone broth

Trust me, bone broth IS worth the hype, especially for fertility.

In Traditional Chinese Medicine, bone broth has been used as a medicinal food for centuries. In China, bone broth is actually known as 'longevity soup'.

When I was given my infertility diagnosis at forty-three, I had swung between being a vegan, vegetarian and pescatarian since I was eight years old. Ironically, I was told by my eldest that I made the best roast chicken ever, even though I had never tasted it. That famous roast chicken was my first introduction to bone broth.

When I first spoke to my functional medicine practitioner about trying for another child, he suggested that I would benefit from upping my levels of protein and that, to do so, I could start incorporating meat into my diet. The thought of it actually made me want to gag, but I decided it was now or never. However, eating even a small amount of red meat was a huge step for me, and one I wasn't ready to take, but then he explained to me the benefits of bone broth and how it helps the gut and supports the uterine lining. Would I be happy to try that out? I thought that, if I could hide it in my food, I could.

So, after our Sunday lunch roast chicken that I'd never tasted, I began to strip off all the meat and simmered the bones overnight and all the next day. I admit, I had to open all the windows in the kitchen because the smell made me feel sick. I have grown to love the smell now; there is something wholesome about it, and it makes me feel grounded in my bones, pardon the pun.

How to make Liberty's naked homemade bone broth:

When making my bone broth at home, I like to keep it simple. In general, after a roast organic chicken, I will strip the carcass of the meat and put the carcass in the fridge overnight. Next morning, as I work from home, I will pop the bones in a cast-iron casserole dish and fill it with filtered water to just under the brim. I'll then simmer it on the hob from seven in the morning till five at night. I do not add any herbs, spices or apple cider vinegar, only a little pink Himalayan salt and black pepper. I make it naked because I can then use it as a base for any soup or curry, and even smoothies, or my otherwise veggie buckwheat muffins that I share with my little girl for breakfast.

Around four or five o'clock, I will then strain off half the broth and use it as a base for our family soup that evening. Then I refill the dish with more filtered water and simmer till bedtime. Then I decant the broth into glass jars for storing. Usually, my jars are empty coconut oil jars, no plastic Tupperware for me, and hopefully not for you either by now! I will keep two or three jars in the fridge, because the broth will last around five days refrigerated. The rest will go into the freezer, where it can last up to twelve months. However, mine doesn't last in the freezer for longer than ten days because I use it in so many dishes and baking. Another storage hack is to pour some of the bone broth into ice cube trays (you can get silicone and stainless-steel ice cube trays from a number of stores). This way, especially in the cooler months, I can pop an ice cube of bone broth into a mug, add some boiling water, some cinnamon, cardamom, whatever floats my boat that morning, perhaps some ginger and a squeeze of lemon, and drink it first thing on an empty tummy to start my day off already on a win. It's also great to have as a warm shot before each meal, if you can, to prep the gut for the food to come.

Making your own bone broth may not be for you; it wasn't for me at the beginning. If not, there are now a number of bone broths out there on the market that are great, be it chicken or beef. However, ideally go for one that is from outdoor bred, grass-fed animals and/or organic, because you want to be consuming the best of the best where you can. Remember I said you are what you eat has eaten? This is so very important in the case of bone broth.

It's also amazing for your skin, because it's full of collagen, and if you have it daily, in a matter of weeks you will not only feel the difference, but see it, so it's a double win.

If you're a vegan or vegetarian, you can have vegetable broth, but it's not the same, and it's not as nourishing because it's missing certain amino acids. Sorry.

Intermittent fasting

The one thing I must stress is not to do intermittent fasting (IF) while trying to conceive. This is because while it is great for things like mental clarity and losing weight, it can be a lot of investment to make sure you meet your nutritional needs within a small eating window, plus it can put a high level of stress on the body, and stress is not good for you and your fertility journey.

Also, if you were to intermittent fast as a woman, you would need to do so in accordance with your menstrual cycle so as not to negatively affect your hormones. This takes a lot of focus and discipline, and at the moment you need to invest your focus in other areas. This is a nurturing time, not a time to place added stress on the body. In addition, when fasting, it's harder to fulfil your protein and healthy fats quota which is needed to support your hormones, as most likely you would only be committing to two meals a day.

Chaps, remember you have hormones too, and we need those swimmers to be fed properly so they can swim not only fast, but in the right direction too! So, the same applies to you gents: no intermittent fasting unless you are clinically obese. Do not worry, though: if you do this properly and eat in line with your fertility needs, you will maintain a healthy weight.

The one difference here between the sexes is I encourage those of you who are female to take your food and drink warm as much as possible, or at least at room temperature. This is because we need to keep the uterus warm.

There are two other ways to warm the uterus through diet. One is through drinking or adding bone broth to your meals and the other is through the wonderful aromatic world of spices.

Seed Cycling for the Ladies

I really like seed cycling because not only does it make you mindful of where you are in your cycle, you can also see how nature supports your female rhythm.

I suggest getting those saved coconut oil jars or nut butter jars out and pre-making your seed mix for each phase of your cycle. We all live busy lives and it takes the stress out of it. You can even label each jar and write a nice message to yourself, so you get a congratulations or a reminder of how great you are each time you reach for the spoon.

Follicular phase (Day 1–14): This is generally when your oestrogen is high. It increases from the day your period starts until the day of your ovulation. This is the phase when you have your pumpkin seeds and your ground flaxseed. A general rule of thumb is a tablespoon per seed. You can add them to Greek, goat or coconut yoghurt, porridge (oat or quinoa or even lentil) and breakfast bars.

Luteal phase (from Day 15 to the start of your period): This is the time when your progesterone is on the rise, as it's after ovulation, when you are leading up to your period, or hopefully your time of fertilisation. Here you have your sunflower seeds and ground sesame seeds.

I like to incorporate these into a bread, pre-made, pre-sliced and stored in the freezer so I can whack it in the toaster and top with avocado or nut butter. But you can put them into a smoothie or on porridge, or you could make some lovely crackers to snack on.

Spices

Now for a few things that truly do smell delightful.

Turmeric

Bright and brilliant, turmeric can help lower inflammation, and we know inflammation in the body contributes to failure of implantation. I like to use fresh turmeric and grate it, but be sure to get your washing-up gloves on so you don't stain your fingers. It's another thing you can add to spice cookies, porridge, smoothies, golden milk and, of course, curries, or you could even take a turmeric supplement.

Cinnamon

My favourite spice, maybe because the smell always reminds me of Christmas. Cinnamon is a powerful antioxidant and great for improving blood circulation. It also helps to balance blood sugar, which many people struggle with. So, if you're trying to step away from sugary sweet treats, putting some cinnamon in your porridge, in your muffins, in your smoothies, in your curries or in your herbal teas, will help with your sweet tooth.

Food Plan

This is simply a sample guide. I tend to work around clients' personalised needs and preferences.

Sunday (prep day)

Spending an hour or so in the kitchen on Sunday will help prepare you for the week.

Ladies, think of where to throw in your seeds this week – chia puddings, overnight oats, breakfast muffins, protein balls.

Boil your bones to make a soup or base for a curry, then freeze the soup and curry sauce to use later in the week or when you have a busy day. You can add your chosen protein on the day. The best way to defrost the sauce is by placing the container in a bowl of hot water. Make your favourite gluten-free bread and some protein balls with mixed nuts, nut butters, protein powder and lashings of coconut oil. You can go wild with the flavours. I make blondie ones that are more nut- or seed-based and even add chilli to my cocoa ones with some Himalayan salt, which are my personal favourite. Once I have made a batch, I freeze them and eat them straight from frozen for that melt-in-the-mouth moment, plus I eat less that way too.

Liberty Mills

As a busy mum, I'm a huge advocate of cook once and eat twice, so you'll see this menu plan uses lots of leftovers!

Ladies, I really would like you to have a warm breakfast a few times a week at least. You could make it and pop it in a flask if you have to take the train or tube to work or are one of those people who like to get to work early and eat there. Just do not eat at your desk. Your meals contain nutrient-dense ingredients to support and balance you in all the right areas. For this to happen efficiently you need to chew slowly and mindfully and not wolf down a sandwich in one hand while typing with the other.

Start with a little cup of bone broth every morning. If you have an outdoor area, gift yourself the time to drink it outside and listen to the birds and connect with nature before you plug into the digital world.

Monday

Breakfast

2 eggs (whichever way you like them) with two sorts of leafy greens sautéed or you can pop in an egg and a few leaves of spinach in a ramekin and pop this in the oven when in the shower. If you are short on time, grab a breakfast muffin or couple of protein balls, etc., but please, please try to carve out 10 minutes for simply being with the food.

Lunch

Soup with the bone broth you made yesterday on prep day with lots of veggies and leftover chicken. You could add beans, lentils or quinoa for extra protein.

Snacks

A chia pudding.

Cucumber, celery, mangetout, sugar snap peas and a tablespoon of cottage cheese.

Dinner

Trout traybake with lots of green veggies.

Evening

A turmeric moon milk.

Moon milks are great to wind down the nervous system before bed. They are made with milk or a non-dairy alternative and are a mix of herbs, spices and adaptogens.

Tuesday

Breakfast

Two slices of homemade gluten-free bread with avocado or nut or seed butter.

Liberty Mills

Snack

Seed crackers and avocado, pea and mint dip.

Lunch

Veggie frittata and salad (if not working at home)

+ two dark leafy greens if working from home.

Dinner

Prawn or white fish quinoa and kale bowl with a baked sweet potato and beetroot dip.

Evening

Lavender moon milk.

Wednesday

Breakfast

Oat crackers and two tablespoons of full-fat cottage cheese and some blueberries or a kiwi.

Lunch

Leftovers from last night's dinner with more GF bread and seed butter or avocado, pea and mint dip.

Dinner

Beetroot and feta patty burgers with sweet potato wedges and homemade slaw.

Thursday

Breakfast

Poached fruit. A great one to add your spices and your seeds to. Choose fruits with a P (fruits with a P make you Poo): plums, prunes, peaches, pears and dark berries too. Add to porridge or chia pudding or overnight oats, with a teaspoon of ghee and cinnamon, and maybe add some grated apple and grated carrot for sweetness.

Lunch

If at home, a chickpea flour wrap with salmon or chicken or mixed beans and a herb salad and tahini.

If not at home, have the filling of the wrap with some oat crackers or flaxseed crackers, or roasted pumpkin.

Snack

Protein balls or 2 squares of dark chocolate (70%-plus cocoa solids and emulsifier free).

Dinner

Chicken/turkey/bean casserole with butterbean tahini mash and greens.

Evening

Saffron milk

Friday

Breakfast

Homemade granola – ladies, you can make this with warm cinnamon milk.

Lunch

Moroccan spiced lentils with kale and amaranth (you can use amaranth like rice).

Snack

Roasted spiced chickpeas.

Celery and cucumber, small palmful of nuts.

Dinner

Thai curry with your choice of protein and your choice of wild rice, quinoa, amaranth or cauliflower rice, sprinkled with kale chips for extra crunch.

Evening drink

Shatavari, ghee and fennel moon milk (have a few hours before bed, as fennel is a diuretic and I don't want you up all night going for a wee!).

Saturday

Breakfast

Green beans and 2 poached eggs, plus a green smoothie.

Lunch

Steamed cod, salmon or poached chicken – your choice – with an artichoke, spinach, asparagus and lentil salad.

Snack

Three dates sliced open with organic thick tahini.

Dinner

Chickpea flour, buckwheat, sweet potato or cauliflower base pizza with kale chips and a garden herb salad.

[Chickpea flour is very versatile, with 20g of protein per cup. Add one espresso cup of water and one espresso cup of chickpea flour to a bowl and whisk into a batter. Pop a tablespoon of coconut oil in a frying pan, add the mixture and cook it as you would a pancake. Use it as a wrap or add toppings and make a pizza.]

Evening drink

Cinnamon, cocoa and turmeric hot chocolate with your choice of milk.

Sunday

Breakfast

Buckwheat pancakes with cottage cheese and berries or coconut yoghurt or full-fat Greek yoghurt.

Lunch

Quiche with broccoli and harissa cannellini beans (slice the leftovers into single servings, wrap in baking paper and freeze for emergency lunches or dinners next week).

Snack

Protein balls.

Fruit and nuts.

Dinner

I'm from the North of England so for me it always has to be a roast chicken with Yorkshire puddings (homemade and gluten free), with roast vegetables, Brussels sprouts and butter bean tahini mash.

There has to be pudding on a Sunday!

I like individual crumbles, so I make them in small ramekins for portion control, with a buckwheat, coconut sugar, ground almond and butter crumble topping. You can make a few and play with the fruit base, pop berries in some, simply slice up apples for others. These can easily be frozen for those rainy days when you simply want to take the weekend off.

Or try Jasmine Hemsley's buckwheat banana bread. It's a part of life in our house, plus it's totally refined-sugar-free, as the only sugar comes from the bananas. And like all baking in our house, we eat half that day and then slice and freeze the rest to be toasted the week after. I have topped this banana bread with anything from avocado to tahini and even beetroot. If you're entertaining guests, family, or friends, you could even make an avocado-sponge cake with almond flour and coconut sugar.

Happy cooking.

'Changing our diet to one which is now balanced, easy to prepare and tastes good has had a significant impact on mine and my husband's health and wellbeing, not just our fertility. Between the two of us we have lost 4 stone which is fantastic in itself, but more importantly we have changed our bodies from the inside. I am no longer pre-diabetic, my blood results show that any deficiencies I used to have are now gone and my severe eczema has vastly improved, supported by the inflammation markers in my bloods now being in the normal range. This I have not seen in years!

'At forty-two I am now the healthiest I have ever been, the quality of my eggs has improved, and I now finally feel that my body is prepared to conceive and have a successful pregnancy. Tackling the demons of a poor diet, in my view, is essential to the turmoil of fertility.'

Amy

Week 11. The New Kids on the Block

Bring on the new wave of fertility treatments!

By now you have well and truly cleaned up your act. You have cleaned up your mind, your body, your daily routine. The way you talk to yourself, talk about yourself and how you talk to others about your fertility journey. You have cleaned up your past, cleaned out your cupboards, overhauled your meals, and your house is now free of chemicals. Gosh, you have been busy, so give yourself a hug. (We need four hugs a day for survival, so there is one, have another from me, now it's only two to go.)

You have laid the foundations for not only your fertility fitness but also your longevity fitness, so when you do meet your child-in-waiting, you will be a happier human and better able to parent them. (And will be that parent who secretly enjoys a play gym just as much as your toddler. You know me by now. I *am* that parent. I do love a slide and ball pit.)

Now is the time for me to geek out and introduce you to the New Kids on the Block. This was one of the first chapters I completed for the book. And it is one of my favourite topics. Yes, I love nineties boy bands, and that's how I see these new treatments – fresh and full of energy. They are all about keeping you young, full of vigour and smiling on the inside. These treatments are the big guns that can help improve the quality of your sperm and the quality of your eggs and keep that uterine lining happy for the most important guest. Yes, these new therapies truly have 'the right stuff' (I couldn't resist it, ha-ha).

Note: The cost of these therapies does range from around the cost of an acupuncture session to several hundred pounds. So, I do understand that not all of these will be accessible to everyone.

HBOT

Hyperbaric oxygen therapy isn't just for the rich and famous. And it's not just for anti-ageing. You may think of rock stars or Michael Jackson sleeping in his chamber and think it's whacky, but no, bear with me. HBOT is one of the best non-invasive treatments around. It's now on the radar of everyone whose optimum physical fitness is a priority (and that is YOU!).

Think about how sports stars, such as boxers and footballers, where an injury could not only cost them the fight or the game, but their future, need to repair their bodies quickly. You too may need to repair your body quickly and HBOT could be your answer for this need for speed. A hyperbaric oxygen chamber looks sci-fi, but it really isn't; it's working with one of nature's life sources – oxygen.

I was introduced to the benefits of hyperbaric oxygen therapy a few years ago by a young female scientist I had befriended on Instagram. She encouraged me to meet a doctor from the Middle East and interview her on the benefits of this treatment for fertility in London, so off I trotted. Before our meeting, the doctor in question flooded my inbox with medical research on the benefits of HBOT on fertility. The data was so compelling I was hooked. I now have clients who regularly use HBOT for long Covid, infections, injuries, marathons and after operations. The benefits are vast.

What does it do?

It breathes life into you on a cellular level. Please note that when choosing your chamber, avoid soft chambers, as all clinical data has come from trials where people have been exposed to oxygen in a hard-shell chamber. All the studies that have resulted in better pregnancy rates have been conducted in hard shells with a pressure of 2.1 to 2.3. So do look for a clinic that has a hard shell and always ask what pressure the chamber can reach. If you are female, it is also important to plan your sessions of HBOT, as it is recommended to start from day 2 to day 5 of your cycle, then break post-ovulation until your next bleed, in case you are pregnant.

There are different-sized chambers, so if you are not a fan of confined spaces, you still have options. There are also different ways of receiving the oxygen while in the chamber, so it is worth ringing around clinics to ask for your preferred way of taking it. One way is a traditional mask that goes over the nose and mouth, another uses tubes up the nostrils. Those with sinus issues may not like this, as it can build up pressure in the sinuses and the cold air can feel like it's stinging. Then there is the one where a tube goes around your neck, almost like a headset with a mic, and the air tube sits under your nose.

The therapy session is the perfect opportunity to take time out. In a single-person chamber you can lie down, plug in your earphones, meditate or listen to your favourite podcast or album. The first time I went to one, I was a little apprehensive as the practitioner closed the lid, even though there was a huge window for me to look out of. My fears of feeling claustrophobic were unfounded, however. I actually fell asleep and woke up feeling refreshed and looked like I had just had a facial. When I came home that evening, my partner even accused me of having Botox.

There are also dual chambers where you can go in with your partner and kick back and watch a movie. Or you can go in with a friend, if he or she is going through fertility issues too perhaps.

How does the oxygen chamber work?

It's easy. You simply lie in there or sit there and you're given pure oxygen to breathe. As the chamber is pressurised to a level that's greater than the normal atmospheric pressures, this increase in pressure allows the oxygen to infiltrate the body's fluids and reach the tissues that can sometimes not be accessed. This in turn encourages the growth of new blood vessels and improves blood flow to those vital areas, including all of your organs, which of course includes your reproductive organs. So, not only does it improve your sperm or your egg quality or, even, your embryo quality, but it also improves your overall health. Normally, each session lasts between 60 minutes and 90 minutes, and it is encouraged that you partake in these sessions several times before planning your conception or egg retrieval.

When arriving at a clinic before your session, make sure they go through a full health check before you enter the chamber. This is so the medical professionals can verify that you are eligible for the treatment. It is important to go to a clinic where there are registered medical professionals such as doctors and nurses, as you can feel a little bit dizzy, or there could be mild discomfort in your ears. The pressure in the ears and head can be similar to when you're taking off or landing in an aeroplane or going for a drive up in the mountains or hills. Where I live, my ears always pop when driving over the moors. If this does occur in the chamber, you'll have a little intercom between you and the medical professional, and they can adjust the pressure so that you can feel more comfortable and at ease.

The high-pressure oxygen also improves your immunity, which is very important for females when trying to conceive, because whilst the body may be trying to fight an infection or some kind of inflammation, it's less likely to get busy with making a baby. So here is a place where we can lower the inflammation and also reduce oxidised stress within the body, which plays havoc with our hormones, therefore lowering our chances of conceiving. So it really is a great thing to try. HBOT is about rejuvenation, replenishing cells and tissues, and repairing them too. It's very relaxing, and a good option for those who are perhaps scared of needles and don't want to go for acupuncture.

Why is it great for women?

Embryo quality and uterine-lining quality can often be contributing factors to the failure of implantation and early miscarriage. Implantation will only take place if the blastocyst is of the best quality and in the best environment, so this is where HBOT can improve two areas in one go. With some women perhaps having scarring as a result of past pregnancies or corrective surgery, this will also help to encourage the healing of those areas.

Having a higher flow of oxygen will improve the blood flow inside the ovaries and this has been shown to increase egg quality. Remember, we can't increase the number of eggs, but we can improve the quality of the eggs you do have, as well as the health of the body that the eggs are developing in and that the embryo will implant into. HBOT is especially beneficial for women who have polycystic ovary syndrome (PCOS) and endometriosis, as these conditions are often linked to inflammation, which is known to negatively affect your chance of fertility. HBO therapy reduces this inflammation and therefore gives you a greater chance of success. It's also a brilliant therapy for those who have autoimmune issues such as rheumatoid arthritis as well as gut imbalances.

One very interesting and important factor regarding hyperbaric oxygen therapy for women is that it can potentially increase the number of eggs produced during a natural ovulation. This can be really helpful for women who have a low harvest when going for IVF preparation. If this is you, try HBOT a good few months before your harvest is scheduled.

Why is it good for men?

HBOT forms new blood vessels in the penile shaft and positively impacts the mitochondrial function of the sperm. Let's rewind all the way back to Week 1, when we got to grips with sperm analysis. Let's shine the spotlight on sperm motility once again. How are they swimming?

Many men over the age of thirty-five have sperm that is not moving towards the egg. They can be immotile, swim zigzag or they can simply vibrate, but they are not in the race to fertilise the chosen egg. Research states that there is a significant decline in motility from the average sperm peak at age twenty-five. This motility further declines by over 50% between age thirty-five and fifty-five. But don't panic if you are reading this and have just turned thirty-six or are even knocking on fifty. Remember, the sperm renews and there is a lot you can do to coach the new batch to go faster and in the right direction. By now I know you are already doing so much and hopefully you are feeling the benefits of the things you have removed and replaced into your life. Perhaps people are commenting on how well you look. Trust me, those sperm are renewing well for when they are next called upon. The great news is that HBOT has an immediate effect on sperm motility. Results of improvement of the motor activity (motility) is reported as soon as 30 minutes after one session of HBOT.[51] This is a great therapy for men to partake in around the ovulation window.

Studies show that HBOT can improve not only motility but morphology too and improve the concentration by decreasing DNA fragmentation. With DNA fragmentation of sperm often being responsible for failure of implantation and early miscarriage within IVF, it's important to look into this area of improvement before entering any type of conception.[52]

IVF outcomes are greatly affected by poor morphology, so if finances permit, I highly recommend investing in a full HBOT protocol before your IVF round if your morphology falls below the Kruger scale of 4% minimum. This is where I do take umbrage with IVF clinics that take clients' sperm with percentages as low as 1%, not enlightening the couple about what this could mean regarding DNA fragmentation and implying that all will be fine due to ICSI. Science says this is most often not the case.

When so much can be done to improve sperm by just 1% or 2% to get them up to the 4% marker of the Kruger scale, it makes sense to explore all areas before depositing the sperm in the vagina or off at the IVF clinic.

The pH level of sperm plays a pivotal role in determining its ability to swim (having that motility rate) and reaching its destination. Think of it as the satnav system for sperm, guiding them towards success. This is where hyperbaric oxygen therapy can be a game-changer. By helping to balance the pH of your sperm, HBOT is like giving those little swimmers a boost in the right direction. Not only does it enhance their motility and velocity, but it can also elevate your HOS score – a crucial measure of sperm vitality and integrity.

Treatment cost:

Most treatments in the UK are anything between £55 and £125 pounds per session, which is 60–90 minutes. Depending on where you live in the United States, it can be around $200–500 and, as with anything you can get a reduction when you buy a bundle of sessions in one go.

Glutathione

One supplement to explore is glutathione. I have a regular IV of glutathione with vitamin C (even though I'm not trying for a baby), because it's good for my body and keeps inflammation low.

Glutathione is a powerhouse antioxidant, but unfortunately it depletes as we age and we are exposed to a multitude of toxins and oxidative stresses.

What is it? Made in the liver, glutathione is the single most powerful antioxidant your body produces and recycles. Glutathione also helps preserve other antioxidants. By adding more into your system, you will boost the body and replace naturally what has been depleted by living a modern stressful life. It also helps to prevent further damage to important cellular components. This is a great one for people who are dealing with an overload of heavy metals and need to support their liver.

How do you take it?

Glutathione can be taken as a supplement orally, by IV or as an injection. When taken orally it's a liquid that you swish around in your mouth. This, apparently, is absorbed into the system by nanotechnology; however, the research is out on whether your body can absorb enough this way to make the difference you want and need. There are many conflicting papers on the subject. Personally, I have tried many glutathione supplements and they taste so disgusting that they are binned after the second go (and I can drink some pretty unpalatable things in the name of health and wellbeing).

This disparity of support for oral administration may be due to the fact it's not normally taken with a high dose of vitamin C, as it would be when taking it intravenously or intermuscular. Plus, if you take a large dose of vitamin C orally, it would have to go through the digestive tract and likely upset the tummy. High doses of vitamin C taken orally can in fact be used to sort out a bout of constipation.

The reason most places combine the glutathione treatment with vitamin C is that they work together as a team. While the glutathione is setting to work, the vitamin C is the cheerleader and coach pushing it along.

Why for women:

Numerous studies indicate that increasing body levels of glutathione can improve not only egg quality but embryo quality also, thus aiding the implantation process.

Women undergoing IVF benefit from increased glutathione as it improves oocyte quality and fertilisation rates.[53]

One 2014 study showed that with higher levels of glutathione, women produce healthier and stronger embryos.

Another study found that, for women undergoing IVF, higher levels of glutathione in their follicles translated into increased fertilisation rates.

Why for men:

Most research on glutathione and male factor infertility is on motility. However, some studies reveal it also has an effect on the DNA. And remember many weeks ago that I asked you chaps to go get checked for a varicocele? There is a study consisting of infertile men with unilateral varicocele or genital tract inflammation where glutathione led to significant improvement in sperm quality.[54]

The great thing about a glutathione IV is you will likely not need more than one to two sessions.

Cost of investment per session: £185–250

Red Light Therapy

Another great new kid on the block is red light therapy. Lots of the clinics that offer HBOT will also have a red light therapy room. Red light therapy is great for both men and women. Because we spend a lot of our time indoors (especially now we're working from home more), we are experiencing less interaction with natural light and movement. Red light therapy enhances our blood flow and circulation.

This is another regulator of women's hormones, which is often a factor in the failure of conception. So, it's another non-invasive way to not only help you relax, but also balance out your hormones to get you ready for your ovulation window. Red light therapy can also reduce oxidative stress.

You can go to a clinic/centre or you can buy a red light wall for your home.

Cost of sessions: £40–55

Cost of a wall at home: £250-plus

The next group are hard for a dyslexic like me to pronounce, never mind write, so I've stuck with the acronyms! But they are creating a stir not only on the fertility circuit but with health practitioners looking at metabolic health and biological health. Let me introduce you to the supplements that are targeting age reversal as well as replenishment.

NAC (N-acetylcysteine)

NAC is a powerful antioxidant that has gained attention in the field of reproductive health. It has been studied for its potential to improve fertility outcomes, particularly in women over the age of thirty-five who may face additional challenges when trying to conceive. NAC works by increasing the production of a molecule called glutathione (you now know what that does). If it were a game of chess, glutathione would be the knights protecting the eggs (queen) and the sperm (king) from oxidative stress (all those pawns). Remember I said I hated oral glutathione, and the scientists are not in agreement if it even works? If a glutathione IV or an injection push may not be available to you, NAC may just be your answer, as you can take it in a capsule and it's much lower cost.

NMN (Nicotinamide Mononucleotide)

NMN is a molecule that has been gaining attention in the field of fertility. Many fertility supplement suppliers are now adding this to their ranges. NMN is a precursor to NAD+, a coenzyme that plays a crucial role in cellular energy production and DNA repair. It's DNA over and over again, isn't it! Once again enforcing this core importance of quality and not simply quality.

As we age, our levels of NAD+ naturally decline, and this decline can negatively impact fertility. That's why I get trolled daily about having children as an older woman. As I always explain, it's not just about our age but the metabolic and biological age of the body that is the true indicator of health, longevity and fertility. I have clients come to me in their late twenties with the metabolic age of a forty-year-old, thus proving we can't rely on the number of candles on the cake to tell us the whole truth.

It's important to note that scientific research on NMN and infertility is still ongoing, and individual results may vary, so test it out and see how your energy and clarity improve. I know that my clarity and energy vastly improve when taking NAC and NMN together. This book, after all, is about providing you with information on what is out there and different ways that you can support yourself, so you can then be empowered to make your choices and create your own bespoke toolkit.

LDN (Low-dose naltrexone)

Chaps, you can skip this one, as it's just for the ladies at the moment. But don't worry, you have some solo sections coming up. I won't forget you, don't forget the stats jump around with their numbers but it's near enough neck and neck a male factor of why I wrote this for you. LDN was brought to my attention by one of the clinics I work closely with. I then delved further into the work of Dr Phil Boyle in Ireland, and the results he has seen with LDN in his fertility practice.

LDN is not like any of the other suggestions above, as it is not something that naturally occurs in the body. Therefore, many in the 'wellness' industry are not in favour of it. However, I am an integrative health specialist and I believe in combining science and nature to help and support people on their wellbeing journeys. Also it's my job to introduce people to what's out there, not to prescribe, but to educate and empower so people can make their own educated choices and also ask questions of their medical teams.

Therefore, due to the potential positive effects of LDN on

women's fertility over thirty-five and those using IVF, I felt it would be remiss not to include it in this section.

LDN is an emerging treatment that has gained attention in the medical community, and I believe in years to come it will be more commonly used. Originally it was used to treat addiction, but it is now being explored for a wide range of conditions, not just infertility but autoimmune issues too. This drug needs to be prescribed, and you can't get it over the counter or at your local wellbeing centre unless it is prescribed by a medical professional who has a licence to do so. People may be apprehensive to use it because of its association with addiction use, but low-dose naltrexone itself does not cause physical or psychological dependence.

With many of us dealing with high inflammation in the body and inflammation having a role in failure of implantation and early miscarriage, this is where LDN comes into play. LDN is believed to modulate the immune system by increasing endorphin levels and reducing excessive inflammation in the body. Therefore, LDN may help create a more receptive environment for conception. To my mind, the host body environment plays just as important a role in fertility as the quality of the egg and sperm.

On that note, LDN is also linked to aiding ovarian function. It is believed to improve blood flow to the ovaries and therefore potentially enhancing follicular development.

Gosh, NAC, NMN, LDN ... they sound more like nineties rock bands than boy bands!

I hope you are beginning to see that, yes, there are many factors that contribute to the decline in fertility; however, there are many viable options out there to reverse the damage already done and protect your future and your child's too.

> 'I tried HBOT for the first time last winter. I live in a cold place in the world and circulation is low and my job and life at the time was high stress. To be honest I had never heard about it before! It has been a nice surprise because immediately after the first session I felt a different wave of energy in my body, calm but energised, but what really impressed me was the mental clarity – the lightness in the head lasted for many days, and my sleep improved.'
>
> Nicole

Week 12. Let's Go 360

My logo has evolved over the years to reflect more about the work I do. It started off as a leaf, which I know seems very predictable for a health coach . . . though the leaf is in the shape of an L for Liberty. The leaf is symbolic of the healing process, about how I encourage people to reconnect to the natural rhythm of life, to nature. But something didn't feel quite right about it.

As my work evolved and I primarily had people coming to me for fertility coaching, the leaf no longer seemed to represent the people who were my core clientele. I was discussing this with a client of mine, and they offered to draw something for me. And they got it, but I think they got it, the representation of imagery in art relating to this process, because they had worked with me for twelve weeks. They presented me with a leaf with an enso circle around it.

The enso circle is a Japanese Zen symbol that is hand-drawn in one or two uninhibited brushstrokes and this is used to express a moment when the mind is free to let the body create. How poignant that was for me, but even before I knew what it represented, I could feel it . . . 'To let the body create.'

When they showed me the 360 unfinished circle, I knew that it represented everything that I believe this work stands for. Not only can a circle be divided up into twelve parts (your twelve weeks), but the circle is present so often in nature too. It's the first thing you may see when you look into a flower, where the petals often arrange themselves in a circular pattern, and this circle is at its heart. Or look at the annual growth rings within the trunks of trees, each ring representing a year of growth.

The enso circle is often drawn with a gap in it, just like mine. This gap symbolises the presence of absence and fullness all at once. This unfinished gap or opening represents the idea that perfection is completely illusionary, and that's what I want people to feel, that there is no perfect fertility journey. That there is still so much beauty and so much to learn from an infertility journey in and of itself. And that even when it comes towards the end, with a birth, an adoption, a surrogacy, whatever it may be, we still keep evolving and moving.

The gap also represents the idea that nothing is a period. Think of the black curve in the circle as the 80% investment in your bio-individuality, and the gap as the 20% where you chill out re the whole thing. No one is going to do *everything* in this book, because even spread over twelve weeks it can be a lot to take on board. And to be honest, I wouldn't want you to do everything and be Perfect Pete or Perfect Penny. Why would a health coach and author say this? Because I want you to take from this what serves you and what benefits you, and for you not to obsess or judge yourself if you don't do this or that. Because guilt and stress are the worst things for your endocrine system, for fertility and for your overall happiness and well-being. Take from it what resonates with you, then go back to Week 1 and see what *has* helped you on this journey and build on it. But if you eat a slice of Bakewell tart (my personal favourite) that isn't refined-sugar-free (yes, even I sometimes eat refined sugar, especially if it's in a cherry Bakewell), don't judge yourself. I'm teased every time I go to the gym that I must be a member of the only gym that serves homemade cakes and afternoon tea. Do what I do, though: say to yourself this is one day out of the week or the month, and it's all the other days that count, not this day. I don't think you would judge me, so please don't judge yourself. Vitamins L and A are the most important vitamins of them all: Love and Acceptance.

I think by now you've heard enough from me (though I encourage you to reach out to me on social media or through my website, so we can share our stories and so we can grow as a collective and bring forth this life of fertility). So I now want you to hear more from people like you. These people surrendered themselves to this work. It wasn't always a metaphorical walk in the park for them, but they did their work and had the happy ending I hope in time you come to have too.

Just like you, they have been through these weeks and all kinds of emotions and transformations along the way. We have cried; yes, I have cried too, normally off camera after a session or in a voice note after a breakthrough. We have also laughed. But most of all we have connected. In a world of fertility that can often be so immensely isolating, having a connection and a voice, I believe, is vital.

So over to these beautiful humans as they share their unfinished 360 circle.

With huge gratitude, I would like you to meet two of my amazing, wonderful, trusting fertility clients.

Pete and Catherine (couple in their forties)

I was so nervous about asking them to do this interview, as I know fertility is still so taboo and I could not take it as a given that anyone would share their stories with me, especially when they had been on such a rocky road. When they sent a voice message saying 'absolutely yes', I cried, as I knew even with this one conversation it was another door opened for someone else.

Liberty: Hi, Catherine and Pete, thank you for doing this. Fertility for you was a bit of a journey, wasn't it?

Catherine: We tried for four years and thought, each year, maybe this isn't our year, and then finally went down the IVF route due to my age. It was there we assumed we would find our answers. When you start asking the doctors why is this not happening? What's going on?, you start realising that actually they may not have the answers. The only answer we got was that it's unexplained infertility.

Liberty: That is pretty much what a lot of my clients get told – unexplained infertility.

Catherine: And so you get to that point where you start going, hold on a second. So actually, when we think about relying purely on medicine, Western medicine, and I'm not dissing medicine – I think it's doing incredible things – but you start realising that they look for just specific things in infertility and there is no holistic approach. They don't look at the entirety of your body as a woman, they don't even look at the entirety of you as a couple. You know, it's almost like they do a test for men and if it's OK, then the whole shift goes onto the woman.

Liberty: What brought you to this work in the book, in asking for help?

Catherine: I came across you on Instagram and I started following you and listening to the things that you said. Much of what you said was addressing those questions I had. It sort of felt like you were attacking the problem from lots of different angles, whereas before it was kind of like the approach to IVF was, just do the IVF and sort of hope it works, that sort of thing. But with your work, we could do that and IVF and that gave me hope.

Liberty: Peter, how was the fertility journey for you?

Peter: Well, I think, ironically, the most impactful thing for me actually doing this work wasn't directly the fertility, it was my gut, wasn't it? And now I know that's related holistically, as getting my health right impacted my fertility as well. For me, the most noticeable difference was, after years and years of not being right with the gut and trying different things, such as the FODMAP diet, and the breath test analysis, and none of this really got it back in order, but doing this work on repair with supplements and understanding how stress affected my gut made a massive difference. So that that was that, for me, and it was the thing that had the greatest impact.

Liberty: Pete, in the whole fertility process, natural fertility for assisted with IVF, out in society, where do you think men fit into it all?

Pete: I think Catherine might have mentioned it before, but I definitely think that there is a lot more focus on women, which is not right. In the sense that emotionally, at least, both people are invested, and obviously physically. I know it is far harder for a woman, but I don't think there's a lot of recognition about how men feel when things don't go right.

Liberty: Do you think the weekly check-in sessions helped, as I have set the book up in a similar way to the way in which we worked? Because quite often we're so busy within a fertility journey trying to survive, so we don't even check in with ourselves, never mind with each other.

Catherine: Yeah, it's interesting, because I was talking to someone about it, and I said, it's like a war, you know, this kind of fertility journey. It's like war, because you've got to have so much resilience. You go into this battle and you don't know whether you're going to come out alive or not. Of course I mean metaphorically, but sometimes kind of generally too, what state will your mental health be in? And then it was funny, because the other person said, well, actually it is like that. Because it is literally life and death. You are battling for life, you are striving to bring life into this world.

Liberty: And often there is death in the battle. If your embryos don't grow, it's a death of that embryo. I was just saying to a client this morning, you know, we are often given the space to mourn a miscarriage, but there seems to be no space to mourn an embryo and this must change.

So, the good news is that the work we prepared for you and that you invested in has worked.

Pete: We try not to get ahead of ourselves, because we've got the scan next week.

Liberty: So how many weeks are you now?

Catherine: Almost thirteen.

Liberty: Will you tell your child you had IVF?

Pete: Personally, I don't think there's any reason not to. Catherine, do you agree with that?

Catherine: Yeah. I mean, I haven't explicitly thought about it, but I think it's only a yes.

Liberty: I think that sometimes, when people don't, it's because of this prejudice that surrounds different routes to a family, but at the same time it contributes to it. Because if we don't say we have had these struggles and took many routes, then what?

Infertility is on the rise and, if we don't talk about it, we are not educating the coming generation. In keeping infertility a taboo, we are exposing them to the trauma that we had to go through. We need to bring these conversations forward and tell our sister, brother, cousin, our children, and educate them, because of this rise of infertility, that neither natural nor assisted fertility is a given.

I miss you guys.

Sam: We miss you too.

Catherine: Come see us.

Now over to one of my very first fertility mummies.

Hannah

Hannah had been recommended to me by a relative who was a medical professional who I'd done some training with. He suggested that she work with me because I would look at her unexplained infertility from perhaps a different angle. I'm sure Hannah won't mind me mentioning that John, her husband, was a little apprehensive at the beginning, but I instinctively knew, after our first Zoom call, that I could help her. So, I was a little thrown when a few days later she replied with an email saying 'thanks but no thanks', and that her husband didn't think it was the right thing for them at that moment in time. But something in me knew she would be back when she was ready. And just as I predicted, a few weeks later I got another email asking for another Zoom call with them both this time to ask a few niggling questions. I suggested that they work with me for three weeks and then after that, if they didn't feel the work was making a positive difference to their life, we would go our separate ways. Hannah started the work the following week, then we hit the three-week mark, and she was in! And as the weeks rolled on, John would jump on the calls too.

Over to Hannah:

Liberty: Hey, Hannah, how old were you when I met you four years ago?

Hannah: I was thirty-four and I'd been struggling to conceive. I had been married for ten years, we'd built our home, our life, and we just were not getting pregnant. And a relative recommended that we reach out to you as a fertility coach. It's something I hadn't heard of before, but it was when I started to talk to you that I realised that I wanted to invest in myself, and it was very clear to me when I finally decided to do the work that I not only wanted a child, but I wanted to invest in myself, and somehow I was putting that off while I was focusing on having a baby.

What doing this work did for me was almost take my mind away and the pressure off conceiving every month, and I learnt slowly to look at what was working for me in my life and what was not working for me or John. I realised that my mum was my mum and I wasn't her mum, and to stop trying to parent her and let her mother me. I had never thought of nutrition as being more than food, like it isn't as simple as opting to make a smoothie or a salad. The biggest one for me was my relationship to my family, to my work.

Liberty: Yeah, that was a struggle at first for you. I remember that, and even at one point you changed jobs while we were working together.

Hannah: Yeah, I did, and I started investing more in my creativity.

Liberty: Yes, you painted me that beautiful card, I still have it on my desk. Hannah, what was the most challenging aspect of our work together?

Hannah: It was creating that discipline that was something I felt, socially, wasn't a thing. It wasn't what people were doing that I knew. I had to invest, to be invested and to help myself, and it was about not just helping my day-to-day, but helping my soul.

And in the end, it was not at all about a pregnancy. It was about me finally coming into being because, when I worked out that, I finally found myself.

Liberty: So where are we at with things now, four years later?

Hannah: I have two great little ones. When we told everyone we wanted another, they said it would take time, but it worked the first time we tried. And I believe, for me, I know everyone's different, but it was because of all this, all this work – I didn't stop. Once I had my first daughter, I continued. And for us, it's become a way of life. It's no longer about fixing our fertility. It's become about who we are, who we are as a family. And I realised, if I can solely look after myself, and show myself all this love, in all these ways, I'm able to look after the other people that I love too.

IVF

This section may not be for everyone, but I feel I would be remiss not to include it in light of the increase in people using IVF on their fertility journey. Also, it's not an actionable week that I do with my clients until we have done all the prep. This is what comes about more often than not further down the road for some or is interwoven if clients come to me with their IVF already booked in.

I was surprised at first to see in my work that many people walk into IVF not knowing what is what, what choices they have, what questions to ask and what emotions are frequently experienced, even though, of course, every experience, every round is different. This applies to both NHS and private IVF.

But first let's acknowledge the grief of the 'natural conception'. Because more than likely there is a degree of loss by the time you get to this stage.

Time after time clients come to me already in the throes of grief. Many women cry for the first session and well into the second and third sessions, as they finally have a safe space to express their emotions. Many are mourning; this can be past pregnancies that were terminated or embryos that never made it to the implantation stage. But what is universal is that they are all mourning the loss of what they expected to be a natural conception and what they thought was a human right to naturally conceive.

Add this to other losses, such as miscarriage, lack of embryo blastocyst development and failure of implantation. This loss of natural conception in isolation can make a person feel betrayed by their own body, angry at themselves, angry at the past or silently or overtly angry at their partner. People often ask me, 'Why me? What did I do wrong?'

It's that prevailing thought that this new path of IVF somehow makes them different from other women and men that they see in the world, in their workplace, in their friendship groups, even within their own family. 'Everyone else can get pregnant, why can't I?'

Here I would like to note that often we don't know what someone else's fertility journey has been, precisely because fertility struggles are still mostly a hush-hush subject. When we see someone walking down the street in their third trimester, we all too often assume that it 'just happened' for them. But we don't know how long they were trying, how many miscarriages they've had, what medications they have been on, what operations they have had to go through. Was it egg donor? Was it sperm donor? Because for some reason there are still so many negative connotations around anything but natural conception.

There is prejudice too. Judging people for being too old, too young, too career-minded, not maternal enough – the list of unwelcome and unsolicited judgements goes on. We often don't speak of them, but we are most certainly all too aware of them. This goes for men as well as women.

For women, the gravity of loss is magnified and distorted by the media. Remember those mirrors in the funhouse at the fair? They are often called crazy mirrors, the ones that reflect your image, only it's not the real you, it's distorted. This is what I feel the image of the 'natural woman', the 'mother' is like in the media. This image of 'woman' and 'mother', what it is to be female, is subliminally entrenched in us from an early age, with fairy stories, schooling, language and sex education. The role of contraception and prevention of pregnancy is heavily laid at the female door, the same with termination. We (the woman) are the gatekeepers to fertility and therefore it is our responsibility. Then, when we are NOT getting pregnant, it is also our failure and our responsibility.

Even Mary the mother of Jesus, the most famous mother of all, had an immaculate conception. She didn't struggle, it just happened by an act of God. She was the chosen one. Many people come to me from all different religious backgrounds and it's common for them to express that they question if their infertility is a sign of them not being dedicated enough to their religion.

It's not just institutions, but advertising, art and especially historical art that all perpetuate this image of the 'natural mother' and 'Mother Earth'. The image of what a woman is is entrenched in fertility. Paintings of women with swollen bellies in 'pregnancy art'. Yes, 'pregnancy art' is a thing, an actual term in the art world. Historically, married women were often in some stage of pregnancy their entire adult life until their menopause, so even when we go to art galleries, these images are imprinted in our subconscious. When we learn art or history in school, images of women are more often than not of pregnant women or women with their child.

This subliminal belief of what a woman is born to be is often carried like a huge weight, especially into the IVF process.

Why have I discussed this in the book? Because I think it's important to address this and say it's OK not to feel OK and understand the contributing factors as to why you may not feel OK. Then we can start to quieten the negative voice and turn up the volume of the woman and man who embrace their own road. Because you can make this journey beautiful and fun too. My wish with this book and my work is to paint a new picture of what a fertility journey can be.

By the time most couples or singles get to the point of IVF, they've most likely been on some kind of journey (I'm often the end-of-the-road person). Hopefully, the practices suggested in Week 9 around investing in self-love and investing in the couple have helped to dilute this feeling of betrayal of the body for not being able to conceive naturally.

So even though we are at the end of the book, please do keep up those practices from all the previous weeks, as it's a journey and we need to tweak and adjust as we go along, especially once we reach the IVF process.

How to De-clinicalise Your Fertility Journey

I'm not a doctor but to me this is the whole point of this book and what I do with my clients, and why they have their breakthroughs, and why many finally meet their child-in-waiting.

I'm not here to dictate historical protocol. This book was birthed because of the demand, from clients, friends, family and the social media world, for knowledge about what can be done to optimise fertility alongside the medical procedures and medications. It's about what you can do to support your body, to support IVF, to support your endocrine system, your sanity and your relationship with each other, yourself and the process. That is where this book and these twelve weeks take their space in your hands. When so much is out of your control, I hope you are now on your way to not only re-humanising your fertility journey but making it your own. Why not make your IVF journey as personal and romantic and as playful as possible.

'We didn't conceive on our honeymoon.'

'It wasn't a romantic weekend away.'

'It wasn't my birthday, anniversary, Mother's Day, Father's Day, my dad's birthday.'

Many couples who have conceived naturally look back fondly at the memory of how it happened on a romantic holiday, a night after a concert, in the back of a car in a field with a picnic. Well, good on them, but it didn't happen like that for most people and they still love their children and their child still loves them. It certainly didn't happen for me like that. I was in immense pain from huge abdominal swelling and, in fact,

I said, 'Don't look at me, just get it over and done with, as I'm never going back to acupuncture again.' Not romantic – painful and hideous, yes, but not romantic – and I wasn't even having IVF. But after the deed was done, I played music, sang with my legs up against the wall and chatted to the child I longed for to extend my family. I made a shitty experience pretty.

I believe that there is not only power in language, but power in thought and perception. If we approach something as a default, that it wasn't what we wanted, going into the process like it's a booby prize, it's going to feel like it. I'm perimenopausal and in no way trying for a child, but every day I take thyroid medication – it's a hormone pill. Every day I take supplements to enable me to thrive at fifty. I'm doing this to replenish what is depleting in my body for the goal of longevity, and so even though I may be the oldest mum at my daughter's primary school, I'm still the fun one who plays and runs around with all the kids and is not trashed at the end of it. I do this with glee, with a vision of what I am investing in. I know it's hard to invest emotionally in IVF, because you don't want to get your hopes up, but it can be a long process, so it would be nice to make it as pleasurable a journey as possible, seeing as you are on it anyway.

Imago therapy

Often because of our love for others, be it our parents, friends or even our partner, we isolate and minimise our own feelings and don't share them because we want to protect them. Because of this, we can bottle things up and then blow up seemingly over nothing. This can create tension with couples during the IVF process. I want to ask you to give yourselves permission to be vulnerable and say it's OK not to be OK. My aim with my clients, and with you, as you are also my wonderful clients, is to break up those clouds and create a blue sky. I encourage you to truly communicate. One practice that is absolute gold where this is concerned is imago therapy. The great thing about it is it's free and you don't have to go to a counsellor to try it.

Imago therapy is an approach that focuses on creating a safe space for partners to truly listen (note it says listen, not talk; listening here means without already wanting to have your say or fix things or diminish or brush them away, and is such an important part of communication) and empathise with one another.

IVF is a highly emotionally charged experience that requires sensitivity, vulnerability and mutual understanding. Imago techniques encourage partners to take turns speaking and listening without interruption, mirroring back what they've heard to ensure true understanding. This slows the conversation down (and the heart rate) and creates space for the deeper feelings that are beneath the IVF journey to be expressed and validated, rather than brushed aside.

So how do you do it?

I like to advise my clients to set the same day and time each week when they know they have this safe space to express themselves. I suggest also using a timer at first so that whoever is speaking doesn't run away with things. Two to three minutes for each person is usually sufficient, so the whole thing is 10 minutes maximum. This stops the practice snowballing into hours of conversation. I also suggest you do it before one or both of you have an activity, so you can't let it drag, like after dinner, before the gym or on a Saturday morning after breakfast before meeting with friends.

Here is an example:

Jane: 'I'm so scared that this IVF cycle is going to fail again. I don't know if I can handle the disappointment.'

Mike: 'OK, let me reflect back what I just heard. You're feeling scared that this IVF attempt won't work out, and you're worried about how you'll cope with the disappointment if that happens.'

Jane: 'Yes, that's exactly it. The failures have been so hard on me emotionally. I just want this to work so badly.'

Mike: 'I can understand why you'd be feeling that way. The ups and downs of IVF must be really draining and you want this so badly.'

Once this is complete on both sides, what I also like is for each person to give the other an action that's actionable that week to help them. It can be as simple as, 'Please make me the first coffee in the morning because that makes me feel seen.' Or 'If I'm angry, please ask me if I am hurting about something.'

Examples of actions:

'I would like two days a week that are IVF-talk-free days, please.'

'Please don't tell your parents about all the IVF appointments – maybe we can update them at certain points?'

'Please find me some smoothie recipes, as the IVF drugs made me so dehydrated last time.'

It can be anything, but it's something to make the other person feel they have one small actionable thing that they can do that will make you feel seen, heard and more secure and safe.

The key elements here are the reflective listening, the validation of feelings, the emphasis on providing emotional support rather than trying to 'fix' the situation, and the simple actionable action to make that other person feel empowered.

I have suggested this work and practised it within sessions with couples, and more often than not they had no idea the other one felt that way. It's a regular safe space for men especially to have a voice, as often, socially, men don't have a safe space or an open place to talk about their fertility journey and how they feel about it all.

Create your own theme tune

> 'Where words fail, music speaks.'
> Hans Christian Andersen

Music can be the most romantic thing in the world.

My first date with my youngest daughter's father was a Coldplay concert. Now, as much as I'm not a huge fan of Coldplay (sorry, Chris Martin and the band), every time I hear one of their iconic songs it makes me feel romantic about what we created from that first date.

If you are as old as me, which you are most likely not, you would have made playlist tapes when you were younger. Now it's all digital, it's even simpler to curate your own. You can make collaborative ones on Spotify or Apple Music and you don't even have to be in the same place to add your chosen music.

I want you to start by creating a playlist for the appointments. It can be the same playlist you use pre any bloods, any operations, egg retrieval, the one you listen to pre-transfer and in the two-week wait. The one you play when morning sickness has taken over. Put it back on in labour and listen with reflection and joy when you feed your baby.

Choose music from those happy times together or when you felt strong and alive and playful with life. From the times you felt most uplifted, powerful, unchained and you could only see the bright lights ahead.

I really missed being around my firstborn Sooay, when I was pregnant with her sister. Because I had her at twenty-three, in many ways I feel that we grew up together, as all of my pivotal, shining memories were with her. When I was pregnant with my second, because she was in America, the void felt even wider. So, I created a playlist of all my favourite songs that reminded me of times with her, when I felt like nothing in the world could stop us, the times we jumped up and down pretending to be in a boy band on the sofa, road trips where we sang so much I often missed a turning or two. Boyz II Men, the soundtrack to *Kramer vs. Kramer*, S Club 7, Blue and J.Lo were the soundtrack to my many antenatal appointments. I was a regular visitor to the clinic, with at least two appointments a week, due to my history of lupus and the effect it could have on my heart and Ulani's risk for a hole in her heart, so the soundtrack was a welcome uplift and I even used it in the first three hours of labour.

This is something that you can do with your partner and the memories you have together, or if you're a single parent, you can choose any memories of when you felt supported, uplifted, unstoppable and seen in your life. I think quite often within IVF people can be treated just as a faceless statistic. Little exercises like this put you at the centre of the process.

I have had clients who have done this and when one of them in the couple is having an emotional blip, the other will pop on the soundtrack and they laugh or hug it out. It certainly has come in handy for my clients, especially the men, who, even in the thick of IVF, still can't find the words they want to express, so they let the music do it for them.

Every milestone is a gift

You and all you are going through is a gift to your child-in-waiting, so why not MAKE each milestone, each stepping stone, into a gift? It's scary, I know.

Start making a scrapbook. You can take a picture of yourself on the way to an appointment, the retrieval, the implantation, etc., and put little quotes under each photo you have printed off. Make a physical scrapbook rather than a digital one, as there is something more personal about physically holding it, something more romantic about seeing the words handwritten. Take a photo of your first injection, with a smiley face marking the spot near where you are about to inject or a big love heart or a message to your child written on your belly. Even after you've been throwing up during your first trimester, this is something to treasure for the future, when at times you feel that future is so far away that it may not become yours. Keep marking the milestone until your child is sixteen and then you can give it to them on their birthday. There will be happy tears all round.

Some final tips from me.

Do your research

Choose the right clinic for your given individual circumstances.

If you are reading this in the UK, as I mentioned early on in the book, look at HFEA (although you need to check when HFEA last did its rating, as it may be outdated and new clinics may be emerging) and Fertility Mapper to know your rights and options if going for NHS IVF or privately funded treatment.

Work out what's best for you and your given circumstances and go into any consultation armed with a list of questions of WHY for me/us.

Be prepared

Go into your appointments prepared, especially your initial consultation. If you are in a couple it's a good idea to have one person ask the questions while the other writes the answers. If you are doing it alone, ask a friend or a family member to join and do the note taking. If on Zoom, you could ask permission to record on a note taker or simply take the notes yourself. All too often I have had clients who meet their consultant for the first time and, when I ask what they said, they are unable to recall anything except the proposed start date, even if it's only been an hour since their appointment.

So much is pinned on these appointments that it's too easy for the mind to do multiple marathons during the appointment, which is why it's good for you to have a list of questions compiled beforehand. The act of writing something down can also trigger a further question to bring up at the end. I suggest asking these further questions at the end of your appointment, however, so the conversation does not spiral and you keep to the point.

Here are seventeen key questions to ask at your first IVF consultation.

1. What are the success rates for IVF at your clinic, based on my specific fertility factors? (Within this I would

advise subdividing this down to each stage. Viable eggs, number of embryos, as well as live birth rates.)
2. What diagnostic tests will be performed to determine the cause of the infertility, if any, on both parties (if there are two of you involved)?
3. What medications will be prescribed during the IVF process, and what are the potential side effects I should look out for, and are there any alternatives regarding drug and dosage?
4. If you have had a previous cycle or cycles at the same clinic or different clinics, would they do things differently in regard to your protocol and why; and if not, why?
5. Is there anything you can do now to improve the success of a cycle and would they recommend delaying it until these changes have been implemented, e.g. lifestyle changes, improving sperm quality, lowering or raising BMI, looking at other factors such as inflammation or gut health?
6. How will you monitor my response to the fertility medications?
7. What is your embryo transfer protocol – how many embryos do you typically transfer, and what factors determine this in my personal circumstance and what are the risks involved?
8. Do you offer preimplantation genetic testing (PGT) for the embryos, and what are the benefits and how long

will it take before the results come back and what are your looking for?
9. If we did do PGT testing, in that time while they were being tested, would you recommend doing another round of stimulation and harvesting in case I want to have more children in the future due to my age, AMH or other health factors?
10. What is your policy on embryo cryopreservation and storage?
11. Does your clinic use time-lapse incubation and imaging?
12. How often will I need to come in for monitoring appointments during the IVF cycle?
13. What is your clinic's policy on transferring fresh vs frozen embryos?
14. Will I be seen by the same team for my appointments?
15. Are you open on the weekends and do you have an out-of-hours emergency contact?
16. What is your multiple birth rate?
17. Would you suggest doing multiple collections due to age if we want to have more children later on?

Don't be afraid to look further afield before you make your decision.

There are now fertility shows and fairs where clinics do talks so you can go and ask questions and often meet clinical staff and see why you may choose to have your treatments with them. This is not just nationally – you can meet clinics from all over the world. If you can't make it in person, many private clinics now have evening webinars where you can register for free and submit questions prior to the event that the moderator will present to the clinicians. Usually these questions are answered by the guest speakers, such as professors, consultants and embryologists.

Don't rule out foreign clinics. Some clinics abroad boast the best results and also may have different restrictions to your own country.

The Czech Republic and Greece have become prominent destinations for international patients seeking IVF treatment. Many of my clients, after failed rounds in the UK, go to Greece or Prague especially and have success. This is largely due to the more permissive regulations around IVF in these countries compared to many other parts of Europe. Factors like fewer restrictions on donor eggs/sperm, surrogacy, and treatment for single women or same-sex couples make Prague and Greece attractive options for patients who may not be able to access certain fertility services in their home countries due to age or BMI. They may also do further investigations as general practice that are add-ons in the UK, therefore it can be more financially accessible even after the expense of flights. Both countries have also developed strong reputations globally for high-quality IVF clinics and experienced fertility specialists, with success rates often on a par with or exceeding those in more developed fertility hubs.

In addition to the favourable regulatory practices, the cost of IVF treatment in Prague and Greece is significantly lower than in Western European nations or the United States. This makes the procedures far more accessible and affordable and, at times, means people can afford more rounds. These countries also provide a great opportunity for that romance and play that I encourage, as they are holiday destinations and are awash with cultural attractions, historic sites and scenic landscapes, which further boost their appeal, providing a welcome respite during what can be a stressful IVF process.

Will IVF bring me closer to the menopause?

Many women come to me worried about IVF and the stimulation, as they are afraid it will bring them into early menopause. Please do not worry. A mass stimulation is not going to affect it at all. Even if you do a number of egg harvests to freeze, as many of my female clients do, to bank for the future, you are still going to be fine.

The fact that we as females are born with all our eggs for our lifetime, and my daughters' eggs were in my tummy before I even got to hold them, still blows my mind. A foetus early in development has around 6 million eggs! Then, by the time they are born into the world, that number will have decreased to around 1 to 2 million already. By the time that you reach puberty, you have between 300,000 and 400,000 eggs. This decrease is caused by the fact that more than 10,000 eggs die each month before you even start puberty.

In a natural menstrual cycle, only one egg is selected and released, while the other eggs that started to mature within that same cycle become degenerate and are reabsorbed by the body. During an IVF cycle, the fertility medications simply cause more of those eggs that would have otherwise degenerated to instead continue maturing and be retrieved, and numbers of eggs stimulated can be anything from single digits to as many as twenty.

The number of eggs retrieved during IVF is typically only a small fraction of the total eggs available in the ovarian reserve at that time. So, IVF does not reduce or deplete a woman's overall egg reserve, it simply allows more of the eggs that would have gone to waste to be retrieved and used for the IVF treatment. The woman's natural egg reserve remains relatively unchanged after an IVF cycle. I like to see IVF as your best cheerleader and personal trainer carrying those eggs that would have fallen by the wayside to the finishing line.

What to expect

Early on in the book I explained the different types of IVF: natural cycle, mild stimulation and full blown. But what happens in this process?

The IVF medication protocol typically begins with ovarian stimulation medications, which are administered through daily subcutaneous (under the skin) injections. They are small and you can get your partner to do them or do them yourself. Normally it's in the chubby skin bit of the belly. These medications, such as follicle-stimulating hormone (FSH) and luteinising hormone (LH), are designed to stimulate the ovaries to produce multiple mature eggs.

Patients may also be prescribed oral medications, such as clomiphene citrate or letrozole, to further support the ovarian response. In addition to the injectable stimulation medications, patients may also be prescribed supplementary medications, including oral contraceptives, progesterone, and GnRH agonists or antagonists.

These medications help regulate the menstrual cycle, trigger ovulation, and prepare the uterine lining for embryo implantation. It's important to note that the specific medications and dosages may vary depending on the individual's fertility profile and the fertility clinic's protocol. I have known clients even have their protocol changed when their normal doctor has been off sick and a new consultant has taken over. So, nothing is set in stone.

Just like any medications, when we create shifts in our hormones, we can experience side effects. Common ones are bloating, mood changes and headaches. So be prepared. For bloating, look at a prenatal probiotic or do some IVF yoga; for moods, journal and warn people; and there are lots of pill-free ways to tackle a headache such as ginger tea and using peppermint oil on the temples as well as Traditional Chinese Medicine combing. Plus, supporting the body by eating more fibre and hydrating with smoothies and watery foods, such as cucumber, celery and grapes, will all help.

Once the eggs have matured, a minor surgical procedure, the egg retrieval, is performed. This involves using ultrasound guidance to gently remove the eggs from the ovaries. The retrieved eggs are then combined with the sperm (either from the partner or a donor). Then the fertilised eggs are allowed to grow and develop for several days, depending on circumstances, and they will transfer on day 3 or day 5. Then comes the gigantic two-week wait until you take a pregnancy test.

If doing any acupuncture or wanting to do hyperbaric oxygen therapy before transfer or post the two-week wait, always be transparent with your medical team. I think it's important to keep an open dialogue with your clinical team as much as possible, as they can only work with what you tell them.

This is also true with any supplements you are taking. Most doctors are happy for you to take many things, but they may even be able to prescribe a higher dose of something you are taking over the counter. Or a supplement may conflict with a drug you are taking or will be taking. So, remember you are a team. I firmly believe in an integrative approach to fertility and that means transparency.

But most of all, try to make it fun: book in lunches, walks, dinners around your appointments so you don't dwell on and mull over every little thing that was or wasn't said. Play that personalised soundtrack, play your own created meditation from Week 1 and perhaps rerecord for each stage of the IVF. Hopefully in a while you will be recording your own hypno-birthing track too.

Everything you are doing on an IVF journey is the kindest loving thing for your child, so try to reflect some of that kindness and gratitude back to each other and to yourself.

Thank you!

All I have left to say is: thank you. If you have this on audio, thank you for listening to my strange accent and to me trying to pronounce certain words. Thank you for hearing about this book in a magazine, on a podcast, social media, from a friend, your mum, dad or your partner and having the hope and the faith to go out and buy it. Thank you for all you've given to trying new things out, replacing, replenishing, rediscovering in these last twelve weeks, twelve months, however long it took you to get through this book.

Where is the work of Week 12, I hear you ask? The work is to keep the circle going and start opening up a conversation with your partner, a friend, a medical professional, your mother, your father, your MP, yourself.

Perhaps share the work you have done here, share the book with someone else or share your experience with me: I would love to read it.

Shout out to me on Instagram @mills.liberty or TikTok @integrativeliberty. And if you see me on the street, do stop and say hello, as it would make my day.

Because this is why I wrote the book. I believe our 360 is always about paying it forward. And with that, I truly hope you meet your child-in-waiting in whatever form they may come to you.

Liberty

References

My Story

1. Oxford Reference (2024). *chronological age*. https://www.oxfordreference.com/display/10.1093/oi/authority.20110803095611419 [Accessed 21 November 2024].

Week 1. Pre-Work

2. Alcohol Change UK. *Unit calculator*. https://alcoholchange.org.uk/alcohol-facts/interactive-tools/unit-calculator.
3. Raee,P., Mofarahe, Z.S., Nazarian, H., Abdollahifar, M.-A., Mahsa Ghaffari Novin, Mahmoud, S. and Marefat Ghaffari Novin (2023). 'Male obesity is associated with sperm telomere shortening and aberrant mRNA expression of autophagy-related genes', *Basic and Clinical Andrology*, 33(1). doi:https://doi.org/10.1186/s12610-023-00188-w.
4. Ferlin, A., Calogero, A.E., Krausz, C., Lombardo, F., Paoli, D., Rago, R., Scarica, C., Simoni, M., Foresta, C., Rochira, V., Sbardella, E., Francavilla, S. and Corona, G. (2022). 'Management of male factor infertility: position statement from the Italian Society of Andrology and Sexual Medicine (SIAMS)', *Journal of Endocrinological Investigation*, 45(5), pp. 1085–1113. doi:https://doi.org/10.1007/s40618-022-01741-6.
5. https://www.hfea.gov.uk/.
6. https://fertilitymapper.com/.

Week 2. Cleaning Up the Present

7. Domar, A.D., Rooney, K.L., Wiegand, B., Orav, E.J., Alper, M.M., Berger, B.M., Nikolovski, J. (2011). 'Impact of a group mind/body intervention on pregnancy rates in IVF patients.' Fertility and Sterility, 95(7), pp. 2269–73. https://www.fertstert.org/article/S0015-0282(11)00476-6/fulltext
8. Jensen, T.K., Gottschau, M., Madsen, J.O.B., Andersson, A.-M., Lassen, T.H., Skakkebæk, N.E., Swan, S.H., Priskorn, L,. Juul, A., Jørgensen, N. (2014). 'Habitual alcohol consumption associated with reduced semen quality and changes in reproductive hormones; a cross-sectional study among 1221 young Danish men.' BMJ Open, 4(9), pp. e005462. https://bmjopen.bmj.com/content/4/9/e005462.
9. www.reveri.com.
10. https://adamcoxhypnotist.co.uk/.
11. https://www.allencarr.com/
12. Carlsen, E., Giwercman, A., Keiding, N., Skakkebaek, N.E. (1992). 'Evidence for decreasing quality of semen during past 50 years.' *British Medical Journal*, 305:609. https://www.bmj.com/content/305/6854/609.
13. Holmboe, S.A., Priskorn, L., Jensen, T.K., Skakkebaek, N.E., Andersson, A.-M., Jørgensen, N. (2020). 'Use of e-cigarettes associated with lower sperm counts in a cross-sectional study of young men from the general population.' *Hum Redprod.*, 35(7), pp. 1693–1701. https://pubmed.ncbi.nlm.nih.gov/32558890/.
14. Moody, O., 'Plea for ban on vaping flavours that harm sperm.' *The Times*, 6 January 2017. https://www.thetimes.com/article/5d127f00-d37d-11e6-962c-fe439ed038d1.
15. Szumilas, K., Szumilas, P., Grzywacz, A. and Wilk, A. (2020). 'The Effects of E-Cigarette Vapor Components on the Morphology and Function of the Male and Female Reproductive Systems: A Systematic Review', *International Journal of Environmental Research and Public Health*, 17(17), p.6152. doi:https://doi.org/10.3390/ijerph17176152.
16. NHS, 'Pregnancy, breastfeeding and fertility while taking or using ibuprofen.' https://www.nhs.uk/medicines/ibuprofen-for-adults/pregnancy-breastfeeding-and-fertility-while-taking-ibuprofen/#:~:text=Ibuprofen.
17. Joshua Rosenthal, *The Power of Primary Food: Tools for Nourishment Beyond the Plate* (New York, Integrative Nutrition Publishing, 2017).

Week 4. Supplements

18. Stanhiser, J., Jukic, A.M.Z., McConnaughey, D.R. and Steiner, A.Z. (2022). 'Omega-3 fatty acid supplementation and fecundability', *Human Reproduction*, 37(5), pp. 1037–46. doi:https://doi.org/10.1093/humrep/deac027.
19. Sprague, M., Dick, J.R. and Tocher, D.R. (2016). 'Impact of sustainable feeds on omega-3 long-chain fatty acid levels in farmed Atlantic salmon, 2006–2015', *Scientific Reports*, 6(1). doi:https://doi.org/10.1038/srep21892.
20. de Roos, B., Sneddon, A.A., Sprague, M., Horgan, G.W. and Brouwer, I.A. (2017). 'The potential impact of compositional changes in farmed fish on its health-giving properties: is it time to reconsider current dietary recommendations?' *Public Health Nutrition*, 20(11), pp. 2042–49. doi:https://doi.org/10.1017/S1368980017000696.
21. Munira, S.M., Lasker, N., Laila, R., Akter, A., Banu, J., Ishrat, S., 'Effect of omega 3 fatty acid in infertile males with oligozoospermia', *International Journal of Reproduction, Contraception, Obstetrics and Gynaecology*, 13(2), pp. 270–6. https://doi.org/10.18203/2320-1770.ijrcog20240121.

    De, C.J., Barratt, C.L.R., Aitken, R.J., Anderson, R.A., Baker, P., Chan, D.Y.L., Connolly, M.P., Eisenberg, M.L., Garrido, N., Jørgensen, N., Kimmins, S., Krausz, C., McLachlan, R.I., Niederberger, C., ÓBryan, M.K., Pacey, A., Priskorn, L., Rautakallio-Hokkanen, S., Serour, G. and Veltman, J.A. (2024). 'Current global status of male reproductive health', *Human reproduction open*, 2. doi:https://doi.org/10.1093/hropen/hoae017.
22. British Nutrition Foundation (2021). 'Vitamin D and immunity.' https://www.nutrition.org.uk/media/1tuj1zrs/vitamin-d-and-immunity_qa.pdf.
23. Aghajafari, F., Nagulesapillai, T., Ronksley, P.E., Tough, S.C., O'Beirne, M. and Rabi, D.M. (2013). 'Association between maternal serum 25-hydroxyvitamin D level and pregnancy and neonatal outcomes: systematic review and meta-analysis of observational studies', *BMJ*, 346, pp. f1169. doi:https://doi.org/10.1136/bmj.f1169.
24. Pilz, S., Zittermann, A., Obeid, R., Hahn, A., Pludowski, P., Trummer, C., Lerchbaum, E., Pérez-López, F., Karras, S. and März, W. (2018). 'The Role of Vitamin D in Fertility and during Pregnancy and Lactation: A Review of Clinical Data', *International Journal of Environmental Research and Public Health*, 15(10), p. 2241. doi:https://doi.org/10.3390/ijerph15102241.
25. Merewood, A., Mehta, S.D., Chen, T.C., Bauchner, H., Holick, M.F. (2019). 'Association between Vitamin D Deficiency and Primary Cesarean Section.' *The*

Journal of Clinical Endocrinology & Metabolism, 94 (3), pp. 940–5. https://doi.org/10.1210/jc.2008-1217.

26. Tamblyn, J.A., Pilarski, N.S.P., Markland, A.D., Marson, E.J., Devall, A., Hewison, M., Morris, R.K. and Coomarasamy, A. (2022). 'Vitamin D and miscarriage: a systematic review and meta-analysis', *Fertility and Sterility*, 118(1), pp. 111–22. doi:https://doi.org/10.1016/j.fertnstert.2022.04.017.

27. Jahan, R.S., Ishrat, S., Shamima Bashar, R., Hossain, M., Akter, S. and Rani, C. (2021). 'Zinc and Folate Supplement Improves Semen Quality: A Prospective Study in Subfertile Males', *Scholars International Journal of Obstetrics and Gynecology*, 4(4), pp. 136–42. doi:https://doi.org/10.36348/sijog.2021.v04i04.010.

28. Hoek, J., Steegers-Theunissen, R.P.M., Willemsen, S.P. and Schoenmakers, S. (2020). 'Paternal Folate Status and Sperm Quality, Pregnancy Outcomes, and Epigenetics: A Systematic Review and Meta-Analysis', *Molecular Nutrition & Food Research*, 64(9), p.1900696. doi:https://doi.org/10.1002/mnfr.201900696.

29. Greco, E., Iacobelli, M., Rienzi, L., Ubaldi, F., Ferrero, S., Tesarik, J. (2005). 'Reduction of the Incidence of Sperm DNA Fragmentation by Oral Antioxidant Treatment', *Journal of Andrology*, 26(3), pp. 349–53. doi:https://doi.org/10.2164/jandrol.04146.

30. Miao, S.-B., Feng, Y.-R., Wang, X.-D., Lian, K.-Q., Meng, F.-Y., Song, G., Yuan, J.-C., Geng, C.-P. and Wu, X.-H. (2022). 'Glutamine as a Potential Noninvasive Biomarker for Human Embryo Selection', *Reproductive sciences*, 29(6), pp.1721–29. doi:https://doi.org/10.1007/s43032-021-00812-y.

31. Ambiye, V.R., Langade, D., Dongre, S., Aptikar, P., Kulkarni, M. and Dongre, A. (2013). 'Clinical evaluation of the spermatogenic activity of the root extract of ashwagandha (withania somnifera) in oligospermic males: A pilot study', *Evidence-Based Complementary and Alternative Medicine*, 2013(1), pp. 1–6. doi:https://doi.org/10.1155/2013/571420.

32. Tais, S. (2014). 'Ashwagandha for Male Infertility', *Natural Medicine Journal*. https://www.naturalmedicinejournal.com/journal/ashwagandha-male-infertility [Accessed 18 April 2023].

33. Nasimi Doost Azgomi, R., Zomorrodi, A., Nazemyieh, H., Fazljou, S.M.B., Sadeghi Bazargani, H., Nejatbakhsh, F., Moini Jazani, A., Ahmadi AsrBadr, Y. (2018). 'Effects of *Withania somnifera* on Reproductive System: A Systematic Review of the Available Evidence.' *BioMed Research International*, 24 January 2018. https://pmc.ncbi.nlm.nih.gov/articles/PMC5833251/.

34. NICE, Joint Formulary Committee (2024). 'British National Formulary (BNF)'. https://bnf.nice.org.uk/.

Week 6. Sleep

35. Kloss, J.D., Perlis, M.L., Zamzow, J.A., Culnan, E.J. and Gracia, C.R. (2015). 'Sleep, sleep disturbance, and fertility in women', *Sleep Medicine Reviews*, 22, pp.78–87. doi:https://doi.org/10.1016/j.smrv.2014.10.005.
36. Mills, P.J., Redwine, L., Wilson, K., Pung, M.A., Chinh, K., Greenberg, B.H., Lunde, O., Maisel, A., Raisinghani, A., Wood, A. and Chopra, D. (2015). 'The role of gratitude in spiritual well-being in asymptomatic heart failure patients', *Spirituality in Clinical Practice*, 2(1), pp. 5–17. doi:https://doi.org/10.1037/scp0000050.

Week 7. Lowering the Toxic Burden

37. Galloway, T.S., Baglin, N., Lee, B.P., Kocur, A.L., Shepherd, M.H., Steele, A.M. and Harries, L.W. (2018). 'An engaged research study to assess the effect of a "real-world" dietary intervention on urinary bisphenol A (BPA) levels in teenagers', *BMJ Open*, [online] 8(2), p. e018742. doi:https://doi.org/10.1136/bmjopen-2017-018742.
38. European Environment Agency (2023). 'Human exposure to Bisphenol A in Europe'. https://www.eea.europa.eu/publications/peoples-exposure-to-bisphenol-a/human-exposure-to-bisphenol-a/download.pdf.static.
39. Sax, L. (2010). 'Polyethylene Terephthalate May Yield Endocrine Disruptors', *Environmental Health Perspectives*, 118(4), pp. 445–8. doi:https://doi.org/10.1289/ehp.0901253.
40. Veeramachaneni, D.N.R., Palmer, J.S. and Amann, R.P. (2001). 'Long-term effects on male reproduction of early exposure to common chemical contaminants in drinking water', *Human Reproduction*, 16(5), pp. 979–87. doi:https://doi.org/10.1093/humrep/16.5.979.
41. ScienceDaily (2024). 'Declining Male Fertility Linked To Water Pollution'. https://www.sciencedaily.com/releases/2009/01/090118200636.htm#google_vignette [Accessed 20 November 2024].

42. Matta, M.K., Zusterzeel, R., Pilli, N.R., Patel, V., Volpe, D.A., Florian, J., Oh, L., Bashaw, E., Zineh, I., Sanabria, C., Kemp, S., Godfrey, A., Adah, S., Coelho, S., Wang, J., Furlong, L.-A., Ganley, C., Michele, T. and Strauss, D.G. (2019). 'Effect of Sunscreen Application Under Maximal Use Conditions on Plasma Concentration of Sunscreen Active Ingredients', *JAMA*, 321(21), p. 2082. doi:https://doi.org/10.1001/jama.2019.5586.
43. Molins-Delgado, D., del Mar Olmo-Campos, M., Valeta-Juan, G., Pleguezuelos-Hernández, V., Barceló, D. and Díaz-Cruz, M.S. (2018). 'Determination of UV filters in human breast milk using turbulent flow chromatography and babies' daily intake estimation', *Environmental Research*, 161, pp. 532–9. doi:https://doi.org/10.1016/j.envres.2017.11.033.
44. Taylor, K.M., Weisskopf, M. and Shine, J. (2014). 'Human exposure to nitro musks and the evaluation of their potential toxicity: an overview', *Environmental Health*, 13(1). doi:https://doi.org/10.1186/1476-069x-13-14.
45. Kazemi, Z., Aboutaleb, E., Shahsavani, A., Kermani, M. and Kazemi, Z. (2022). 'Evaluation of pollutants in perfumes, colognes and health effects on the consumer: a systematic review', *Journal of Environmental Health Science and Engineering*, 20(1), pp. 589–98. doi:https://doi.org/10.1007/s40201-021-00783-x.

Week 8. Cleaning Up Your Home Environment

46. Hernandez, L.M., Xu, E.G., Larsson, H.C.E., Tahara, R., Maisuria, V.B. and Tufenkji, N. (2019). 'Plastic Teabags Release Billions of Microparticles and Nanoparticles into Tea', *Environmental Science & Technology*, 53(21), pp.12300–10. doi:https://doi.org/10.1021/acs.est.9b02540.
47. Ogulur, I., Pat, Y., Aydin, T., Yazici, D., Rückert, B., Peng, Y., Kim, J., Radzikowska, U., Westermann, P., Sokolowska, M., Dhir, R., Akdis, M., Nadeau, K. and Akdis, C.A. (2023). 'Gut epithelial barrier damage caused by dishwasher detergents and rinse aids', *Journal of Allergy and Clinical Immunology*, 151(2), pp. 469–84. doi:https://doi.org/10.1016/j.jaci.2022.10.020.
48. Celebi Sozener, Z., Ozdel Ozturk, B., Cerci, P., Turk, M., Gorgulu Akin, B., Akdis, M., Altiner, S., Ozbey, U., Ogulur, I., Mitamura, Y., Yilmaz, I., Nadeau, K., Ozdemir, C., Mungan, D. and Akdis, C.A. (2022). 'Epithelial barrier hypothesis: Effect of the external exposome on the microbiome and epithelial barriers

in allergic disease', *Allergy*, 77(5), pp. 1418–49. doi:https://doi.org/10.1111/all.15240.

Week 9. Investing in Self. Investing in the Couple. Making Love, Not a Baby

49. van der Kolk, B., *The Body Keeps the Score: Brain, mind, and body in the healing of trauma* (New York: Penguin Books, 2015).

Week 10. Diet

50. Environmental Working Group (2024). 'The invisible threat: EWG analysis shows you could be eating as many as 12 plastic bags a year.' https://www.ewg.org/research/invisible-threat-ewg-analysis-shows-you-could-be-eating-many-12-plastic-bags-year.

Week 11. The New Kids on the Block

51. Jakubik-Uljasz, J., Gill, K., Rosiak-Gill, A. and Piasecka, M. (2020). 'Relationship between sperm morphology and sperm DNA dispersion', *Translational Andrology and Urology*, 9(2), pp. 405–15. doi:https://doi.org/10.21037/tau.2020.01.31.
52. Ozgok Kangal, K. and Ozgok, Y. (2021). 'Assisted reproductive treatments with hyperbaric oxygen therapy in male infertility', *Türk Üroloji Dergisi/Turkish Journal of Urology*, 47(2), pp. 98–105. doi:https://doi.org/10.5152/tud.2020.20328.
53. Adeoye, O., Olawumi, J., Opeyemi, A. and Christiania, O. (2018). 'Review on the role of glutathione on oxidative stress and infertility', *JBRA Assisted Reproduction*, 22(1), pp. 61–6. doi:https://doi.org/10.5935/1518-0557.20180003.
54. Lenzi, A., Sgrò, P., Salacone, P., Paoli, D., Gilio, B., Lombardo, F., Santulli, M., Agarwal, A. and Gandini, L. (2004). 'A placebo-controlled double-blind randomized trial of the use of combined l-carnitine and l-acetyl-carnitine treatment in men with asthenozoospermia', *Fertility and Sterility*, 81(6), pp. 1578–84. doi:https://doi.org/10.1016/j.fertnstert.2003.10.034.

Liberty's Trusted Sources

Further reading

Shannah H. Swan, *Count Down: How Our Modern World Is Threatening Sperm Counts, Altering Male and Female Reproductive Development, and Imperiling the Future of the Human Race* (New York, Scribner, 2021).

Anthony G. Jay, *Estrogeneration: How Estrogenics are Making you Fat, Sick and Infertile* (Tallahassee, Pyrimidine, 2017).

Dr Julie Von, *Spiritual Fertility: Integrative Practices for the Journey to Motherhood* (Hay House, London, 2019).

Services

Find an integrative dentist

British Homeopathic Dental Association: https://www.bhda.co.uk/page3.html

My dentist and a firm favourite of my clients: Dr Shabir Pandor is at 44 Harley Street, London, W1G 9PS (020 7580 1076). He's not too spenny either. I had root canal at the same time as my friend and he was cheaper than her local dentist. His talents don't end with your teeth; he also practises Light Kinesiology and the Biophoton Realignment Mirror work.

Liberty Mills

Wellbeing Centres

HUM2N (a doctor-led biohacking centre)
HUM2N Clinic
35 Ixworth Place
London SW3 3QX
United Kingdom
Telephone: +44 20 4579 7473
Email: concierge@HUM2N.com

The Wellness Lab
21 Knightsbridge
London
SW1X 7LY
Email: info@thewellnesslab.com
Telephone: +44 77 2460 1630

Positive IV
(A clinically led and medically supported integrative clinic based in the North West)
Unit 1, Crown Business Park
1 Cowm Top Ln
Rochdale
OL11 2PU
Email: email@positiveiv.com
Telephone: 01706 582451

Womb massage

Alexa Dean, London: https://alexadean.co.uk/contact/
Nikki Hills, South and London: nikki@nikkihillis.com
Root Medicine, Midlands and London: https://rootmedicine.co.uk/

Find an Acupuncturist

https://acupuncture.org.uk/

Supplements

I don't want to overwhelm you, so here are the basics:

Purer Mama Essence Capsule
(Fertility supplement support)
Founded by an award-winning UK obstetrician, a paediatrician, psychologists and wellbeing practitioners to produce evidence-based formulas.
www.purermama.co.uk

Inessa Pregnancy Multinutrient
Created by Liza Marogy, who also got her own lifelong autoimmune disease into remission.
https://www.inessawellness.com
Omega-3

Bare Biology
https://www.barebiology.com/
CoQ10

Pharma Nord
https://www.pharmanord.co.uk/
Vitamin D with K2

Liberty Mills

Sunday Natural
https://www.sunday-natural.co.uk/

For more in-depth guidance, go to my website and download your free supplement guide sheet for women and men.

Acknowledgements

This book was not just created by me – it took a collective effort to bring it all together.

360 Fertility was born out of my clients and everyone that has asked for fertility advice for a friend or a loved one. As one person, I knew I couldn't reach everyone, but I wanted to. I am so grateful to everyone who has supported me along the way – whether you've sent me a message, followed me on Instagram or trusted me and become a client. This work has come to life because of you.

A huge shout-out to Fay Ward for responding to a message from me at silly o'clock asking for help to find an agent. To Gordon Wise, who saw potential in the project and introduced me to the truly amazing Ciara Finan. Ciara, you are the most wonderful cheerleader.

To Anna Steadman, as soon as I read your email, I knew you were the right person to get this book out there, you just got it. You are the best guide through the publishing world, a space I knew nothing about. Thank you for your patience.

And of course, to Sophie Elletson, who dotted the i's and crossed the t's – your attention to detail was invaluable.

Let's not forget Ben, the best proofreader ever. You helped me make this book clearer and sharper, always asking, 'What are you trying to say here, Liberty?'

And to Jenna, for all those Sunday mornings we spent together as a dynamic laptop duo surrounded by chaos in the play gym. Don't worry, I will still be there Sunday, 9.30am sharp – there's a second book to come!

Index

abortions 112–14
acetylcholine 161
acupuncture 22–3, 153
adaptogens 22, 150, 159
addictions
   dopamine reward 277–8
   health history 41, 46
   LDN (low-dose naltrexone) 322–3
   sugar 90
age, chronological and biological 8, 321
alarm clocks 188
alcohol
   health history 38, 44
   sleep effects 80–2
   zero intake 20–1, 78–85
alcohol ethoxylates 241–2
aluminium 212
AMH (anti-mullerian hormone) 62
anaemia 162
Andrews, David 215
anti-mullerian hormone (AMH) 62
antibiotics
   health history 41, 47
   mother lineage history 48
antidepressants 93–4, 164
anxiety
   avoid ashwagandha 149
   health history 41, 47
ashwagandha 22, 148–50
asparagus 283

asparagus allergies 152
autoimmune conditions
   avoid ashwagandha 149
   HBOT (hyperbaric oxygen therapy) 313
   thyroid function 63
   see also lupus
Ayurvedic medicine
   ashwagandha 148–50
   tongue 75–6

B vitamins
   foods 281, 282, 287–8
   riboflavin (B2) 159
   supplements 163
babies, microbiome 49–50
bath exercise 99–101
bathing 213–14
bathroom cleaners 251–2
bedtime routines 76–7, 182–90
beetroot 284
benzyl acetate 224–5
birth defects, smoking effects 85
birth story, your own 35–6, 42, 48–52
births, past and anxiety 118–22
blackout blinds 191
bleach 249
blood flow
   L-arginine 152
   L-citrulline 153
   red light therapy 319

vitamin D 139
blood sugar levels 90, 296
blueberries 283
BMI, IVF eligibility 35–6
body, reconnecting with 99–101, 267–9
body clock 179, 180
body fat, visceral 37
bone broth 290–3
bowel function 38–9, 45–6, 169, 196
Boyle, Phil 322
BPA (bisphenol A) 206, 209–10, 211–12, 246–7
Brazil nuts, selenium 157
breastfeeding
 immune system 51–2
 microbiome 50, 52
breathing 170–2
Bristol Stool Chart 39, 45
broccoli 282
butternut squash 282

C-sections
 mother lineage history 48–9
 vitamin D levels 65, 138
cabbage 283–4
calcium 159, 284
Cameron, Julia 97
cancer history, avoid DHEA supplements 158
candida 77–8
Castile soap 250–1
cherries 280–1
chicken, bone broth 290–3
chickpeas 282
childhood trauma 115–18
chlorate 204–5
chlorine 201, 246
choline 161–2
cigarettes 85–6
cinnamon 296
circadian rhythm 179, 180
citrus foods 281
cleaning products
 dishwashers 242–8
 surface cleaners 248–53
clothes washing 253–4
coffee 41, 46
collagen 146–8

communication, imago therapy 343–6
contraceptive pills, in tap water 203
cooking, utensils and pans 229–30
cortisol 180, 195–6
counselling 14
cravings 41, 46, 279–80

dehydration 169
dentists 369
depression, men 19
DHEA 157–8
diet
 cheat days 275–7
 eat the rainbow 280–4
 fats 287
 folate 286
 food diaries 272–3
 health history 40–1, 46
 meal plans 297–305
 no fasting 293–4
 planning 278–80
 prebiotics and probiotics 288–9
 protein 286–7, 290
 seed cycling 294–5
 way of living 271–2
 see also foods
dishwasher products 242–8
DNA
 NMN (nicotinamide mononucleotide) 321
 sperm quality 59
dopamine 194–5, 277, 279
doulas, birth trauma 112, 119, 121

earplugs 191–2
Earth children 4
egg donors 11, 14–15
egg quality
 glutathione 318
 HBOT (hyperbaric oxygen therapy) 313
 prescription drugs 94
eggs, ovary selection 69–70
eggs (food) 273–4
eicosapentaenoic acid (EPA) 131
endocrine-disrupting chemicals (EDCs) 207–9, 215–16, 230, 237
endometriosis
 HBOT (hyperbaric oxygen therapy) 313

vitamin D 65, 140
energy levels, health history 41, 47
enso circle 325–7
epigenetics 14–15
epinephrine 194
epithelial barrier 243–4
erectile dysfunction 85, 257
exercise
   hormones 194
   increasing 172–4
   menstrual cycle 172–4
   morning routine 194–5
   toning down 20
eye masks 191

fasting 40, 46, 293–4
fat in the body, visceral 37
fats, dietary 125, 285, 287
ferritin 66
Fertility Mapper 67
fertility meditation 105–8
fibre 282, 283
fibroids 151
fight or flight response 171
figs 283
fish
   cost 131–2
   omega-3 132–3, 283, 284
folate
   compared to choline 162
   foods 281, 283, 284, 286
   men 60–1
   supplements 142–4
   women 64
folic acid 142
follicle development
   alcohol effects 83–4
   collagen 146
   shatavari 151
foods
   bone broth 290–3
   buying local 238–9
   collagen 147
   eat the rainbow 280–4
   fertility foods 289
   growing 239
   hydration 91, 169–70, 288

   meal plans 297–305
   oils 285
   omega-3 131–3
   planning 278–80
   selenium 157
   spices 296
   takeaway meals 276
   tinned 211–12
   UPF (ultra-processed foods) 275, 277–8
   you are what you eat has eaten 273–4
   see also diet; fruit; vegetables
fruit
   clean fifteen 235–6
   dirty dozen 234–5
   washing 232–3, 236, 239–41

genes
   egg donation and epigenetics 15
   folic acid conversion 142
ghee 285
glutathione 144, 156, 316–19, 320
glycaemic index (GI) 125
gratitude journals 77, 97–9, 193–4
Graves' disease 71
Greeks, ancient 196–7
grief, infertility diagnosis 337
grounding 279–80
gut health
   alcohol ethoxylates 242–3
   epithelial barrier 243–4
   history 38–9, 45–6
   importance 53–4
   L-glutamine 148
   maltodextrin 125
   orthophosphate 202
   probiotics 157

H.A.L.T. reasons for sugar eating check 90–1
Hashimoto's disease 63
HBOT (hyperbaric oxygen therapy) 308–14, 324
health, four pillars overview 167–75
health history
   men 41–7
   overview 32–3
   women 34–41

HFEA 66–7, 349
Hippocrates 196–7
homosalate 216
hormones
  acetylcholine 161
  alcohol effects 83
  chlorate effects 205
  endocrine-disrupting chemicals (EDCs) 209–10, 215–16, 222
  exercise 194
  sleep 180, 181–2, 190–1
  sugar effects 90
  synthetic 203
  trauma effects 119
  see also luteinising hormone; oestrogen; progesterone; testosterone
HRT 213
Huberman, Andrew 195–6
hydration 91, 168–70, 288

ibuprofen 92–3
ICSI (intracytoplasmic sperm injection) 69
imago therapy 343–4
immune system
  breastfeeding 51–2
  HBOT (hyperbaric oxygen therapy) 312
  LDN (low-dose naltrexone) 323
  own birth story 49–51
implantation failure
  alcohol effects 83
  range of factors causing 74–5
Indian ginseng 148–50
induction 24–6
inflammation
  gratitude journals 194
  HBOT (hyperbaric oxygen therapy) 312, 313
  LDN (low-dose naltrexone) 323
  leaky gut 243–5
  omega-3 131
  orthophosphate 202
  stress 268–9
  sugar consumption 88–9
  tongkat ali 154
  turmeric 296
Institute of Integrative Nutrition (INN) 19, 97

insulin levels 90
intermittent fasting 293–4
intimacy 255–61
iodine 284
iron 66, 162, 281, 282–3, 284
IVF
  age and chances 14
  appointment preparation 350–4
  choosing a clinic 349, 352–4
  HFEA 33–7, 349
  imago therapy 343–6
  implantation failure 74–5
  menopause 354–5
  milestone scrapbooks 348–9
  music playlists 346–8
  NHS eligibility 35–6
  process and protocols overview 356–8
  starting the journey 336–40
  success rates 74
  types 66–70
IVM (In Vitro Maturation) 69

journalling 77, 95–9, 192–4
joy 37, 43

kidney disease 164
kitchens
  dishwasher products 242–8
  surface cleaners 248–52
  washing up 242

L-arginine 152, 159
L-citrulline 153
L-glutamine 148
LDN (low-dose naltrexone) 322–3
lead in water 201–2
lentils 281
letters of love 101–5
levothyroxine 13
libido
  maca 159
  shatavari 151
  stress 256
  vitamin D 139, 140
lithium medication 164
liver disease 164
love letters 101–5

lupus 18, 22–3
luteinising hormone (LH) 93

maca 22, 158–9
magnesium
  foods 283
  supplements 128
magnesium stearate 124–5
makeup and toxins 222–7
maltodextrin 125–6
massage, navel massage 104
medication, prescription drugs 92
meditation
  childhood trauma 116–18
  fertility meditation 105–8
melatonin 154–5, 180, 191
men
  depression 19
  fertility and being overlooked 16–18, 330–1
  health history 41–7
  initial medical tests 54–61
  refusing to take part, finding the why 114–18
  supplements list 130
  weight 42–3
menopause
  HRT 213
  IVF 354–5
  PFAS 209
menstrual cycle
  exercise levels 172–4
  health history 40
  maca 159
  seed cycling 294–5
  tampons and toxins 218–20
mercury 148
methylene chloride 224–5
microbiome
  alcohol ethoxylates 242–3
  breastfeeding 50, 52
  orthophosphate 202
  own birth story 49–51
microchimerism 114
microplastics 203, 208, 231–2
Mills, Liberty
  clients 3, 27–8, 328–36

logo 325–7
personal story 1–2, 4, 7, 8–16, 18–19, 20–6, 100, 172–3, 341–2, 347–8
training 1, 2, 19, 26
mind
  journalling 95–9
  negative self-talk 98
miscarriage 103, 120–1, 140–1, 160, 210
mitochondria 48
moon milks 299
mother lineage history 34–5, 41–2, 47–9
movement *see* exercise
MRI scans, men 55, 57
MTFHR gene 142
multivitamin supplements 123–4, 127–8
music playlists 346–8
musk ketone 223
myo-inositol 164

NAC (N-acetylcysteine) 320
NAD+ 321
navel massage 104
negativity 95, 106
nervous system, breathing 171–2
nitric oxide 153
NMN (nicotinamide mononucleotide) 321
non-stick pans 230–1
NSDR (non-sleep deep rest) 180
nutrition
  own birth story 47–8
  see also diet
nuts, selenium 157
nylon 232

octinoxate (ethylhexyl methoxycinnamate) 216
octocrylene 216
oestradiol 182
oestrogen
  DHEA 157–8
  sleep 182
  sugar effects 90
  vitamin D 139
oils, cooking 285
omega-3
  foods 132–3, 283, 284
  supplements 130–6

oral health 41, 47, 369
oregano oil 78
orgasm 259–60
orthophosphate 202–3
ovarian function
　alcohol effects 83
　BPA (bisphenol A) 210
　collagen 146
　DHEA 158
　LDN (low-dose naltrexone) 323
　sleep 182
　smoking and vaping effects 87
oven cleaner 251–2
oxidative stress 163, 202, 319, 320
oxybenzone (benzophenone-3) 215–16

painkillers 92–3
palm oil 125
parasympathetic nervous system 171–2
parsley 282
perfume and toxins 220–7
period pants 219
pesticides 233–5, 237–8
PET (polyethylene terephthalate) 206–7
PFAS 209
phones 186–90, 192
phosphates 202–3, 246
phthalates 206, 221–2, 224
plastic 205–6
plastics 205–8, 229–30, 231–2, 246, 276
plums 283
polycystic ovary syndrome (PCOS)
　avoid DHEA supplements 158
　BPA (bisphenol A) 210
　HBOT (hyperbaric oxygen therapy) 313
　myo-inositol 164
　shatavari 151
　vitamin D 65, 140
polypropylene (PP) 232
pomegranate 281
positivity 97–9
PQQ (pyrroloquinoline quinone) 163
prebiotics 288–9
pregnancy art 339
preparation
　health history overview 32–3
　men, medical tests 54–61

men's health history 41–7
women, medical tests 61–6
women's health history 34–41
prescription drugs 92
probiotics 50, 157, 288–9
progesterone 160
protein 286–7, 290
pumpkin 282
pycnogenol 153

raspberries 281
red light therapy 319
relationships
　the £10 date mission 261–4
　dreams and calendar mission 265
　imago therapy 343–6
　intimacy 255–61
　no-fertility-talk day mission 266
　recreate your second date mission 264–5
religion 339
riboflavin (B2) 159
Rosenthal, Joshua 97

sanitary towels 218
Sasse, Stephanie Fine 194
screen time 37, 44, 186–90, 192
seed cycling 294–5
selenium 156–7, 159
self-talk, negative 95
serotonin 190, 194
sex
　bedroom ban mission 266–7
　intimacy 256–9
　orgasm 259–60
shatavari 151–2
shift work 177, 178
showers 213–14
skin-to-skin contact 49
skincare and toxins 220–7
sleep
　alcohol effects 80–2
　children and routines 183–5
　health history 38, 44–5
　hormones 180, 181–2
　importance 177
　irregular patterns 178–81

morning routine 192–7
  sleep hygiene 76–7, 182–3, 185–92
smoking 38, 44, 85–6
soap bags 226
sperm analysis 55
sperm quality
  alcohol effects 82–3
  ashwagandha 149–50
  collagen 147
  DNA fragmentation 59
  endocrine-disrupting chemicals (EDCs) 209–10, 223
  folate 143
  HBOT (hyperbaric oxygen therapy) 314–16
  L-arginine 152
  L-citrulline 153
  omega-3 135
  prescription drugs 94
  shatavari 152
  smoking and vaping effects 85, 86–7
  varicoceles 28–9, 56–7, 318
  vitamin E 145
  zinc 155–6
SPF 214–17
spices 296
stillbirth 25–6
stimulants, sleep compensation 180
stomach ulcers, avoid ashwagandha 149
stress
  infertility journey 327
  inflammation 268–9
  libido 256
  reduction and pregnancy rates 73
  tongue indentations 76
sugar
  availability 21, 89–90
  candida 77–8
  cravings 21, 41, 46, 279
  fertility effects 88
  glycaemic index (GI) 125
  H.A.L.T. reasons check 90–1
  hormone imbalance 90
  inflammation 88–9
sunlight 137, 195–6
sunscreen 214–17
supplements

additives to avoid 124–6
ashwagandha 148–50
B vitamins 163
bioindividuality 129
choline 161–2
collagen 146–8
DHEA 157–8
folate 142–4
food first 127
glutathione 316–19
iron 162
L-arginine 152
L-citrulline 153
L-glutamine 148
maca 158–9
melatonin 154–5
men 130
multivitamins 123–4, 127–8
myo-inositol 164
omega-3 130–6
PQQ (pyrroloquinoline quinone) 163
probiotics 157
progesterone 160
shatavari 151–2
sources 371–2
tongkat ali 154
vitamin C 144–5, 317–18
vitamin D 136–8
vitamin E 145–6
women 129
zinc 155–6
sweet potato 282, 283–4
sympathetic nervous system 171

T3 see triiodothyronine
T4 see thyroxine
takeaway foods 276
talc 125
tampons and toxins 218–20
tea bags 231–2
teeth grinding 76
testosterone
  alcohol effects 83
  DHEA 157
  endocrine-disrupting chemicals (EDCs) 210, 216, 223–4

ibuprofen 93
maca 159
smoking and vaping effects 87
sugar effects 90
tongkat ali 154
vitamin D 139
TG *see* thyroglobulin
TGAb *see* thyroglobulin antibodies
thirst 91
thyroglobulin antibodies (TGAb) 63
thyroglobulin (TG) 63
thyroid function
   avoid ashwagandha 149
   chlorate 205
   endocrine-disrupting chemicals (EDCs) 215–16
   iodine 284
   men 59–60
   sleep 182
   women 13, 62–4
thyroid peroxidase (TPO) antibodies 63
thyroid-stimulating hormone (TSH) 63, 182
thyroid-stimulating immunoglobulin (TSI) 64
thyroxine (T4) 13, 59–60, 62
tinned cans 211–12
titanium dioxide 124
tomatoes 280
tongkat ali 154
tongue
   health indicator 54, 75–6
   indentations 76–7
   yellow coating 77–8
Traditional Chinese Medicine 290
trauma
   hormone effects 119
   infertility diagnosis 268
   past births 119–21
   from your own childhood 115–18
travel and body clocks 179
triclosan 246
triggers, asking for help 112, 113
triiodothyronine (T3) 59–60, 62
TSH *see* thyroid-stimulating hormone
TSI *see* thyroid-stimulating immunoglobulin
turmeric 296

UPF (ultra-processed foods) 275, 277–8
urine colour 169–70
urologists 55–6
uterus
   collagen 146
   diet 294
   progesterone 160

vagus nerve 98
van der Kolk, Bessel 268
vaping 38, 44, 86–7
varicocelectomy 57–9
varicoceles 28–9, 56–7, 318
veganism 293
vegetables
   clean fifteen 235–6
   dirty dozen 234–5
   washing 232–3, 236, 239–41
vegetarianism 293
vernix 49, 51
visceral fat 37
vitamin A 283–4, 285
vitamin C
   foods 281, 282, 283, 284
   supplements 128, 144–5, 317–18
vitamin D
   C-section incidence levels 65, 138
   foods 285
   men 61–2
   requirements 141
   sunlight 137, 195
   supplements 136–8
   women 64–5, 70
vitamin E
   foods 285
   supplements 145–6
   vitamin C 144
vitamin K 285

waist circumference 36–7, 43
waking routines 192–7
washing up 242
water
   bathing 213–14
   bottled 205–8
   filters 199–200
   hydration 91, 168–70

tap water toxins 200–5
watermelon 281
weight
  IVF eligibility 35–6
  recent history changes 36, 43
weighted blankets 190–1
women
  bath exercise 99–101
  health history 34–41
  initial medical tests 61–6
  letter to your mummy 103–4

reconnecting with your body 99–101, 267–9
society expectations of fertility 338–40
supplements list 129
weight 35–7
work-life balance 37, 43–4

yoga nidra 177, 180

zinc 155–6, 282, 283